GnRH ANALOGUES

THE STATE OF THE ART AT THE MILLENNIUM

GnRH Analogues

The State of the Art at the Millennium

A Summary of the 5th International Symposium on
GnRH Analogues in Cancer and Human Reproduction
Geneva, February 1999

Edited by
Bruno Lunenfeld

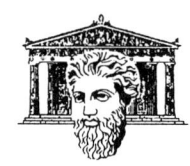

The Parthenon Publishing Group
International Publishers in Medicine, Science & Technology

NEW YORK　　　　　　　　　　　　　　　　LONDON

Cover: Space-filling rendering of the GnRH antagonist consensus model derived from NMR studies of four cyclic GnRH antagonists. Each color is representative of a defined pharmacophore. Calculations and rendering by Steven C. Koerber and Jean E. Rivier (see Chapter 2)

Library of Congress Cataloging-in-Publication Data
GnRH analogues: the state of the art at the
   millennium / edited by B. Lunenfeld
      p. cm.
      Includes bibliographical references and index
      ISBN 1–85070–097–4
      1. Luteinizing hormone releasing hormone—
Derivatives—Mechanism of action.
      2. Luteinizing hormone releasing hormone—
Derivatives—Therapeutic use.
      I. Lunenfeld, Bruno
         [DNLM: 1. Gonadorelin—analogs &
      derivatives.   2. Gonadorelin—therapeutic
      use.   WK 515 G5729 1999]
QP572.L85G56 1999
612.6—dc21
DNLM/DLC   99–33960
   for Library of Congress   CIP

British Library Cataloguing in Publication Data
GnRH analogues: the state of the art at the
   millennium
      1. Luteinizing hormone releasing hormone –
   Derivatives
   I. Lunenfeld, Bruno
   615.7'66
   ISBN 1-85070-097-4

Published in the USA by
The Parthenon Publishing Group Inc.
One Blue Hill Plaza
PO Box 1564, Pearl River,
New York 10965, USA

Published in the UK and Europe by
The Parthenon Publishing Group Limited
Casterton Hall, Carnforth,
Lancs. LA6 2LA, UK

Copyright © 1999 The Parthenon Publishing Group

No part of this publication may be reproduced, in any form, without permission from the publishers except for the quotation of brief passages for the purpose of review.

Typeset by AMA DataSet Ltd., Preston, Lancs, UK
Printed and bound by Butler & Tanner Ltd., Frome and London, UK

Contents

	List of principal contributors	vii
	Preface B. Lunenfeld	1
1	GnRH: mechanism of action C. Gründker and G. Emons	7
2	GnRH analogues towards the next millennium J. Rivier	31
3	The use of GnRH antagonists in assisted reproduction technologies R. E. Felberbaum and K. Diedrich	47
4	Application of GnRH analogues in the management of female infertility E. Lunenfeld	65
5	GnRH analogues: safety aspects K. Bühler	73
6	Current status of medical treatment of sex offenders with GnRH analogues D. Seifert	83
7	Pathogenesis and medical management of uterine fibroids I. A. Brosens and B. Lunenfeld	91

8   GnRH analogues in the management of endometriosis: 99
    K. W. Schweppe

9   GnRH analogues in ovarian, breast and endometrial cancers   105
    S. Westphalen and G. Emons

10 GnRH analogues in the management of prostate cancer and benign   121
    prostatic hyperplasia
    J. E. Altwein

    Index   131

List of principal contributors

J. E. Altwein
Department of Urology
Krankenhaus der Barmherzigen Brüder
Romanstrasse 93
D-80639 Munich
Germany

I. A. Brosens
Medisch Centrum
Tiensevest 168
B-3000 Leuven
Belgium

K. Bühler
Center for Gynecological
  Endocrinology and Reproductive
  Medicine
Lornsenstrasse 4–6
D-22767 Hamburg
Germany

G. Emons
Department of Obstetrics and
  Gynecology
University Göttingen
Robert-Koch-Strasse 40
D-37075 Göttingen
Germany

R. E. Felberbaum
Department of Obstetrics and
  Gynecology
Medical University of Lübeck
Ratzeburger Allee 160
23538 Lübeck
Germany

B. Lunenfeld
Faculty of Life Science
Bar-Ilan University
Ramat Gan
Israel

E. Lunenfeld
Soroka University Medical Center
Faculty of Health Sciences
Ben Gurion
University of the Negev
Beer Sheva 84101
Israel

J. Rivier
The Salk Institute for Biological
  Studies
10010 N. Torrey Pines Road
La Jolla
California 92037-1099
USA

K. W. Schweppe
Ammerland Clinic
Lange Strasse 38
26655 Westerstede
Germany

D. Seifert
Institut für Forensische Psychiatrie der
  Universität/Gesamthochschule
  Essen
Rheinische Kliniken Essen
Virchowstrasse 174
45147 Essen
Germany

Editorial note

Throughout the text the numbers shown in brackets, for example [39], refer to the original abstract numbers as published in *Gynecological Endocrinology*, 13, Supplement 1, 1999 (which was the Book of Abstracts for The 5th International Symposium on GnRH Analogues in Cancer and Human Reproduction).

At the end of each chapter, after the references, a bibliography is provided which lists in full the abstracts quoted in that chapter.

Preface

B. Lunenfeld

Ever since the isolation, identification and synthesis of gonadotropin releasing hormone (GnRH) in 1971, the interest in the application of GnRH analogues has experienced an explosive growth rate. We are finally beginning to understand the molecular biology and mechanism of action of GnRH and its analogues. Furthermore, the major components of the cellular basis of desensitization when GnRH is administered chronically have been delineated. The recent cloning of the human GnRH receptors and elucidation of their sequences have promoted several laboratories to model the GnRH receptor and to use the receptor structure to design more efficient analogues as well as peptidomimetic or non-peptidic orally active antagonists. The state of the art of GnRH antagonist chemistry, pharmacology, preclinical and clinical trials are presented in this book.

The potency of GnRH and its analogues as stimulators or inhibitors of pituitary gonadotropin secretion permitted its exploration as a method of 'reversible medical gonadectomy', applied to treatment of diseases dependent on gonadal steroids. It served as a basis for developing four types of treatment modalities, based on different rationales:

(1) To suppress sex steroids in diseases in which development or progress is sex steroid-dependent (metastatic prostate cancer, hormone-dependent breast and endometrial cancer, uterine fibroids and endometriosis);

(2) To inhibit the precocious appearance of mature-type GnRH pulsatility (central precocious puberty) or delay normal onset of pubertal GnRH pulsatility in order to postpone epiphysial closure and thus permit growth to continue (in slow-growing children);

(3) To control the dynamics of gonadotropin secretion in induction of ovulation or superovulation (as adjunctive treatment of anovulation, polycystic ovary disease and assisted reproduction protocols);

(4) To exploit possible local effects of GnRH agonists on tissues having GnRH receptors (some types of malignancies, uterine fibroids, etc.).

Studies which were reported during the 5th International Symposium on GnRH Analogues in Cancer and Human Reproduction and which are summarized in this volume also indicate that GnRH analogues offer an adjunctive therapeutic modality to gynecological surgery. They can also offer an alternative and successful therapeutic approach to control, quite efficiently and quickly, benign gynecological disorders associated with excessive menstrual blood loss.

The state of the art, the rationale, advantages and pitfalls of the use of agonists for the management of endometriosis and uterine fibroids are discussed in detail.

The top world authorities on prostate cancer management addressed different issues in diagnosis, screening, and prediction of prognosis as well as the intrinsic heterogeneity of the tumor, explaining its manifold response levels which make the therapeutic approach of this complex, life-threatening and painful disease so difficult; all these issues are summarized in this book. There is consensus today that androgen deprivation is the mainstay of hormone-dependent advanced carcinoma of the prostate. Surgical castration, conceived by most men as a permanent and humiliating procedure, can now be effectively replaced by administration of GnRH analogues. During this Symposium, the roles of GnRH antagonists in the management of prostate cancer and benign prostate hypertrophy were discussed for the first time and are reported in detail in this book.

The clinical results of the use of implants and longer-acting GnRH agonists and antagonists were presented and a chapter is devoted to their effects on quality of life and compliance. It was demonstrated that intermittent androgen deprivation, in contrast to continuous androgen deprivation, increased quality of life and progression-free survival, and it was suggested that surgical castration will become just a painful memory of the past. The issue of neo-adjuvant hormonal therapy before radical prostatectomy is also addressed in this publication.

Results of basic and clinical studies with GnRH analogues alone or in combination with antiestrogens in hormone-dependent breast cancer were presented. The culmination of the large ongoing adjuvant program will provide information that will determine if GnRH analogues will enter the next millennium as a new treatment option for early breast cancer.

The first clinical results of the use of GnRH antagonists in patients with ovarian cancer are reported.

PREFACE

In the management of the infertile patient, where conventional treatment regimens have failed, GnRH agonists have been successfully utilized to suppress the pituitary–ovarian axis prior to stimulation of follicular growth and induction of ovulation, concomitantly with exogenous gonadotropins. It is estimated that, in many countries, more than 80% of superovulation protocols include the use of GnRH analogues. The advantages and disadvantages of different protocols and different preparations were discussed in detail during this Symposium and are reported in detail.

Unlike the potent GnRH agonists, whose availability has allowed their widespread use during the past 10 years, the lack of production of suitable antagonists, which work by receptor occupancy, has been disappointing. Antagonists require precise topological features for high binding affinity to the receptor. In the past, the introduction of hydrophobic amino acids in positions 1, 2 and 3, as well as the addition of very basic groups in position 6, to the antagonists have often led to high histamine release from rat mast cells and induced cutaneous anaphylactic reaction-like reactions. The newer generations of antagonists, particularly the latest ones, show negligible histamine release as well as increased solubility and, therefore, really take advantage of the remarkable acute and potent properties. The two sessions devoted to antagonists demonstrated the progress made in this field and show results with some of the newer antagonists in clinical situations. These are presented and discussed in detail.

The reasons for development of GnRH antagonists are discussed at length. The available new GnRH antagonists, their chemical properties and pharmacodynamic characteristics are described, and future developments regarding optimal formulations and chemical structures tailor-made to specific GnRH receptors are evaluated.

The advantages and disadvantages of agonists versus antagonists in future therapeutic regimens are explored. The avenues of future research concerning GnRH analogues (agonists and antagonists) are specified and some particular features are discussed in depth. The ideas presented and discussed in this volume will hopefully permit you to formulate future perspectives for research and applications of GnRH analogues.

It was shown during this Symposium that third-generation GnRH antagonists seem to be potent and well-tolerated inhibitors of the pituitary–gonadal axis in men and women. Preliminary studies have indicated that they rapidly and reversibly suppress testicular and ovarian function in a dose-dependent manner and may be clinically effective and acceptable drugs for the treatment of some gonadal hormone-dependent disorders.

However, it also became evident during this meeting that none of the GnRH agonists or antagonists which were clinically tested were capable of total suppression of LH or FSH.

As always, with any new class of therapeutic agents, safety considerations must be paramount. Potent endocrine drugs such as the GnRH agonists and antagonists should not be expected to be without 'side-effects'. These unwanted effects will include sequelae of their mechanism of action and reflect the induction of a hypogonadotropic hypogonadism.

Relatively new data were presented indicating that the persistence of minimal amounts of GnRH analogues during the luteal phase at the time of implantation seems to have no adverse effects on the pregnancy rate and fetal well-being. Furthermore, data are presented on the effects of GnRH analogues on the trophoblast and embryo and on results following inadvertent administration during early pregnancy. Long-term safety aspects with GnRH analogues in precocious puberty are also presented.

In vitro and *in vivo* effects of GnRH antagonists and their initial safety profiles and hormonal dose–response characteristics are reported.

We discussed in this Symposium and report in this volume whether both the symptoms of the underlying disease and the adverse effects derived from ovarian quiescence can be reliably suppressed by the administration of sub-threshold doses of GnRH analogues, combined treatment of GnRH analogues with low-dose estrogen–gestagen, low-dose estrogen replacement therapy or by combining GnRH analogues with synthetic steroids.

To take stock of the state of the art in this fast-moving field, the 1st, 2nd, 3rd, 4th and 5th International Symposia on GnRH Analogues in Cancer and Human Reproduction have been held in Geneva in 1988, 1990, 1993, 1996 and 1999. These symposia permitted frank interdisciplinary discussions and the exchange of results as well as the development of ideas. The interdisciplinary nature of this field became evident from the 124 lectures presented on the basic and clinical features of GnRH agonists and antagonists during the 1999 Symposium.

For the benefit of the participants and for those who could not join us, these state-of-the-art lectures are reproduced in the form of this book. It is our hope that the chosen rapporteurs have presented in this volume the state of the art of GnRH agonists and antagonists. The book summarizes clearly the manifold impact of GnRH analogues in the management of many pathological conditions and may open new dimensions for students, physicians, biochemists and researchers. We also hope that this volume will stimulate you and your colleagues to join us at the 6th Symposium in February 2001.

1
GnRH: mechanism of action

C. Gründker and G. Emons

INTRODUCTION

The hypothalamic decapeptide gonadotropin releasing hormone (GnRH), also called luteinizing hormone releasing hormone (LHRH), plays an important role in the control of mammalian reproduction[1–3]. It is released from the hypothalamus in a pulsatile manner and stimulates the synthesis and release of luteinizing hormone (LH) and follicle stimulating hormone (FSH). Chronic administration of long-acting agonists, leading to pituitary desensitization, has been used for selective medical hypophysectomy as well as for medical castration in many diseases[1,2,4,5]. Recently, potent antagonistic analogues of GnRH, such as cetrorelix, ganirelix, antarelix, ramorelix and others, have become available for clinical testing[4,5,6] [64, 67, 68]. GnRH antagonists competitively block pituitary GnRH receptors and inhibit gonadotropin release from the start of administration, avoiding the initial increase of LH and FSH secretion and the subsequent transient gonadal stimulation. This stimulation inevitably precedes selective medical hypophysectomy and medical castration induced by GnRH agonists and may lead to flare-up in disease[4,7].

In addition to these well-documented classic hypophysiotropic actions, GnRH might play a role as a modulator of activity in the brain and many peripheral organs[1,4,8–13]. An autocrine/paracrine function of GnRH has been suggested to exist, for instance, in the placenta[14–17], granulosa cells[18–20], myometrium[21] and lymphoid cells[22–24]. In addition, it is probable that such GnRH-based autocrine systems are present in a number of human malignant tumors including cancers of the breast, ovary, endometrium and prostate.

In this chapter, our present knowledge on common features as well as on differences in the mechanisms of action of GnRH in the pituitary, in normal extra-pituitary tissues and in cancers is reviewed.

PITUITARY GONADOTROPHS AND OTHER NORMAL TISSUES

GnRH receptor

GnRH binds to a specific GnRH receptor. Cloning of the GnRH receptor from several mammalian species[10,25–31] has revealed that the receptor is a member of the large superfamily of seven transmembrane domain receptors that binds to G-proteins[10,26,27,32,33]. The GnRH receptor completely lacks a cytoplasmic C-terminal tail, which has been implicated to play a role in rapid desensitization[34]. Upon hormone binding, the GnRH receptor normally acts via pertussis toxin-insensitive G-proteins, most probably belonging to the Gq-family[35]. Through these Gq-proteins, it is probable that phospholipases and calcium channels are activated as the next steps in the signal transduction [19] (Figure 1).

Activation of phospholipases and mobilization of calcium ions

The activation of the inositol phosphate pathway drastically changes the physiology of the cell by releasing calcium ions from the endoplasmic reticulum followed by external calcium ion influx via L-type voltage-sensitive calcium ion channels[36,37]. The most important initiation point of this pathway is a seven-transmembrane domain receptor like the GnRH receptor coupled to phospholipase C (PLC) via Gq-proteins[25,38–40]. When GnRH binds to its receptor, the receptor activates the Gq-protein[35,41–45]. This activation dissociates the G-protein into its subunits, which are then able to activate a set of phospholipases C, namely, PLC-β1 and PLC-β2[46–48]. These two types of phospholipase C can catalyze the hydrolysis of phosphatidylinositol-4,5-bisphosphate (PIP_2) into the two second messengers inositol 1,4,5-triphosphate (IP_3) and diacylglycerol (DAG)[36,37,49]. IP_3 is able to open calcium ion channels of the endoplasmic reticulum, releasing a large store of calcium ions into the cytoplasm followed by an influx of external calcium ions via L-type voltage-sensitive calcium ion channels[36,37]. DAG activates protein kinase C (PKC), which in turn activates the proton pump that exchanges sodium ions for hydrogen ions. The result is the elevation of intracellular calcium ions and an increase of intracellular pH[36,37]. Following a short lag of approximately 1–2 min, phospholipase D (PLD) and phospholipase A_2 (PLA_2) are activated by GnRH resulting in phosphatidylethanol (PE) and phosphatidic acid (PA) production or in arachidonic acid (AA) production, respectively[50–54]. Since PA is converted to DAG by PA-phosphohydrolase, DAG will be produced in sequential phases, initially by PLC and later by PLD, providing a possibility for selective and sequential activation of various PKC subspecies.

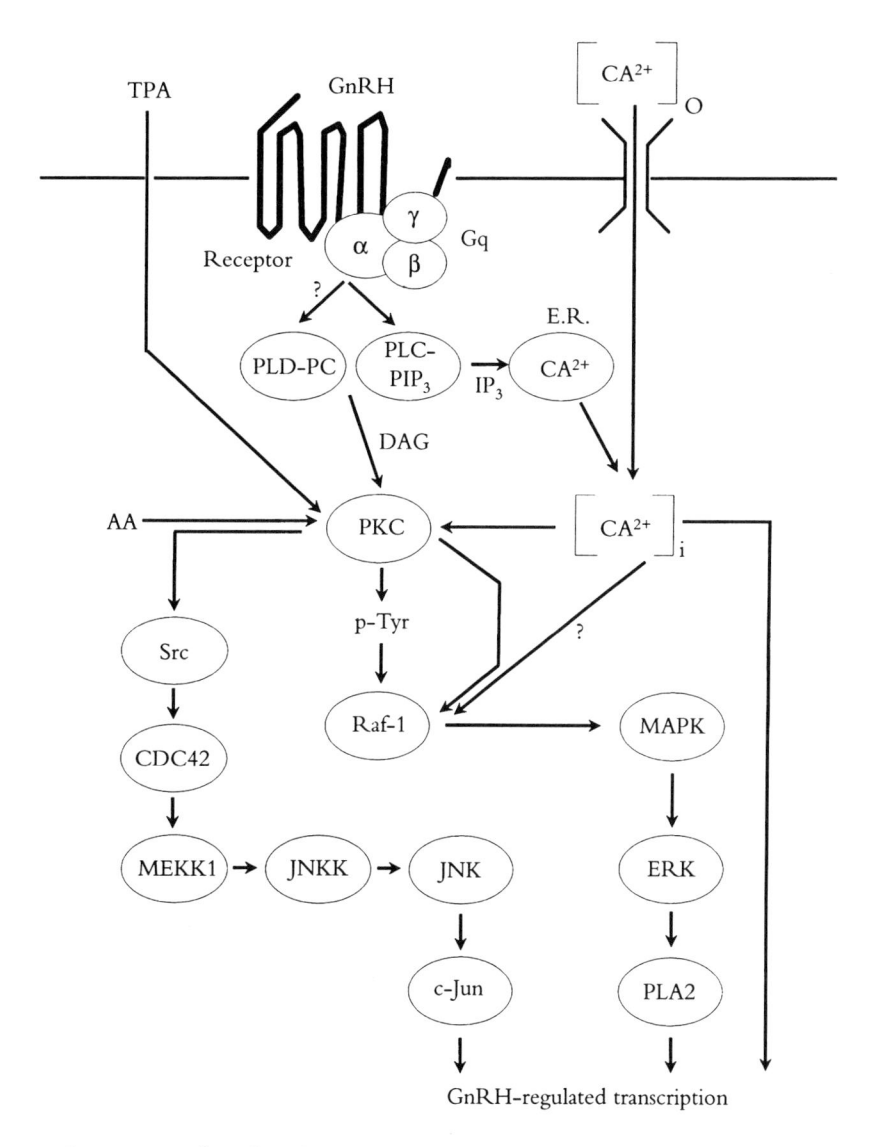

Figure 1 Proposed molecular mechanisms of signalling of the GnRH receptor in the pituitary gland. Modified according to Reiss and colleagues[73] with supplements. For references and further details, see text

Role of protein kinase C

The PKC family consists of a group of at least ten related isozymes which can be subdivided into those containing a calcium ion-binding domain and those lacking this domain which have been shown to be unresponsive to calcium ions[55,56]. The PKC isoforms are classified into conventional PKCs (cPKC: α, βI, βII, γ), novel PKCs (nPKC: δ, ε, η, μ, θ), and atypical PKCs (aPKC: ζ, λ, ι)[57]. cPKCs are activated by calcium ions, DAG and phosphatidylserine (PS). nPKCs are calcium independent and are activated by DAG and PS. aPKCs are calcium and DAG independent and are activated by PS and PIP_2[57]. Pituitary gonadotrophs express PKCα, β, δ, ε and ξ[58]. PKC consists of a C-terminal kinase domain and an N-terminal regulatory domain. The regulatory domain binds and thus inhibits the catalytic domain. A variety of compounds unmask the catalytic domain; these include calcium ions, DAG, arachidonic acid, phosphatidylserine and phorbol esters[55,56,59,60]. Agents that modulate PKC can be categorized into those that influence the catalytic domain and those that affect the regulatory domain[61,62]. PKC plays a key role in signal transduction of different ligands and in different tissues[57,63,64]. Initially, rapid activation of the phosphoinositide turnover by GnRH might provide calcium ions and early DAG needed for cPKC activation[46]. Following a short lag period, GnRH-activated PLD might generate late DAG via PA formation, which might be involved in nPKC activation. Finally, AA, which is liberated by activated PLA_2, further supports selective activation of PKC isoforms together with or without other cofactors[52,65,66]. GnRH-activated PKC is translocated from the cytosol to the membrane. PKC inhibitors reduce GnRH action, and down-regulation of PKC inhibits GnRH stimulation of LH release and gonadotropin subunit mRNA expression[67,68]. Nevertheless, the role of PKC in GnRH signal transduction is still controversial[69]. Findings that PKC is involved in GnRH-induced gonadotropin secretion raised the possibility that protein phosphorylation is positively correlated with gonadotropin release. Protein dephosphorylation is positively involved in GnRH stimulation of gonadotropin secretion, but possibly this site of action is further downstream to calcium ion mobilization as well as PKC activation. PKCα and β are potential candidates for mediation of exocytotic responses elicited by GnRH[69]. Newest results showing that the elevation of PKCβ, δ and ε is mediated by Ca^{2+} and autoregulated by PKC suggest that PKCβ, δ and ε are likely candidates to participate in GnRH actions[70,71].

Role of mitogen-activated protein kinase

Receptor protein tyrosine kinase (RPTK, growth factor receptors) as well as G-protein-coupled receptors have been found to be involved in a sequential activation of a set of cytosolic protein kinases known as the mitogen-activated protein kinase (MAPK) cascade[72]. The MAPK signalling pathway, consisting of members of the serine/threonine protein kinases and their downstream kinases such as ribosomal S6 kinase, is the best defined cascade of signalling via activated kinases. The large number of distinct upstream mitogen-activated protein kinase kinases (MAPKK) and mitogen-activated protein kinase kinase kinases (MAPKKK) provides a cascade that amplifies surface signals and increases the sensitivity of the response. Cross-talk with other kinases, such as PKC, are thought to 'fine tune' networks. The GnRH receptor activates the MAPK cascade via alternative mechanisms involving PKC-dependent or -independent pathways or the βγ-subunits of G-proteins and different potential sites of activation such as Ras, Raf-1, or others[72]. Phosphorylated MAPK is translocated to the nucleus, and leads to activation of transcription factors such as c-fos, initiating cellular responses including growth and differentiation. In pituitary cells GnRH stimulates MAPK, which might be involved in gene expression of the gonadotropin α-subunit. PKC and calcium ion mobilization participates in the activation of MAPK by GnRH, with calcium ions being necessary downstream to PKC[73].

The PKC- and calcium ion-dependent MAPK cascade is also involved in the negative regulation of basal and GnRH-stimulated GnRH receptor transcriptional activation[74].

Role of arachidonic acid

The activation of PLA2 results in the release of AA from cellular phospholipids and in the formation of eicosanoids[75]. Several groups have found that AA and some of the lipoxygenase products are involved in GnRH-induced gonadotropin secretion and gonadotropin subunit expression[36,52,72,75–77]. AA and its products might act by activation of specific PKC isoforms. The leukotrienes formed during GnRH action might be a first messenger in an autocrine/paracrine loop of an amplification cycle during GnRH action[75].

Jun N-terminal kinase pathway

The MAPK signalling pathway is not the only route by which GnRH communicates with the nucleus. Naor's group[78] showed that the Jun N-terminal kinase pathway (JNK pathway) is significantly activated in response to GnRH. The JNK cascade utilizes a sequential activation of p21-activated kinase/mixed lineage kinase (PAK1/MLK), mitogen-activated kinase kinase kinase1 (MEKK1), stress-activated protein kinase kinase1/mitogen-activated protein kinase kinase7 (SEK1/MKK7), and JNK1/2 to activate transcription factors such as c-Jun, AFT2, and Elk 1[79,80]. The GnRH-induced activation of the JNK pathway is much greater than that of the MAPK cascade, but the time course of JNK activation is slower than that of MAPK[78]. The stimulation of JNK activity is mediated by a unique pathway that includes sequential activation of PKC, c-Src, CDC42 and MEKK1[78].

Cross-talk between GnRH-induced signal cascades

GnRH-induced gonadotropin synthesis and secretion is mediated through complex cross-talk between calcium ion mobilization, PKC subspecies, AA and its metabolites, and the MAPK pathway[81]. During exocytosis calcium ions and PKC act in parallel and exert an additive influence upon gonadotropin secretion[68,70]. During GnRH-induced transcription of the gonadotropin α-subunit and PKCβ genes, calcium ions and PKC act sequentially in a non-additive manner. GnRH-induced LHβ mRNA elevation is mediated by either calcium ions or PKC but not by both messengers, since the combined activation of both pathways results in inhibition of LHβ gene expression[52]. GnRH-induced FSHβ mRNA elevation is mediated by PKC alone, since calcium ions were found to be inhibitory. Differential cross-talk of calcium ions and PKC is involved in the diverse effects of GnRH upon gonadotropin secretion and synthesis[49,81]. It is possible that different PKC isoforms such as calcium ion-dependent or -independent PKCs are involved in the diverse GnRH actions. Furthermore, the steroid hormones progesterone and estrogen exert modulatory effects on the GnRH receptor signalling pathway[82–90].

GnRH receptors in normal extra-pituitary tissues

In normal human extra-pituitary tissues, including breast, placenta, ovary and testis, controversial data have been obtained relating to the presence of GnRH receptors[8–10]. Northern blot analysis failed to detect GnRH receptor mRNAs in any of the non-pituitary tissues examined[27]. However, using the reverse transcriptase-polymerase chain reaction (RT-PCR), these mRNAs were recently identified in granulosa–luteal cells[19].

In the ovary, GnRH receptor mRNA expression is under both homologous and heterologous regulation. GnRH up-regulates the steady-state levels of its receptor, while LH/human chorionic gonadotropin (hCG) exerts a negative effect on GnRH receptor expression in granulosa cells. The GnRH receptor is regulated tissue specifically and the effects of GnRH support the role of GnRH as an autocrine regulatory system in the ovary, in addition to its well-established function as a neuroendocrine regulator at the level of the anterior pituitary gland [20].

Koch and co-workers [21] demonstrated that GnRH mRNA is expressed in the mammary gland of pregnant as well as lactating rats. Further bioactive GnRH was found in the milk of different species including the human. In virgin, pregnant and lactating rats, GnRH receptor mRNA expression was also found, identically with that of the pituitary receptor. Only low-affinity binding sites were found. However, GnRH treatment did not result in activation of adenylyl cyclase or MAPK, whereas adenylyl cyclase could be stimulated by forskolin, resulting in increased cAMP levels, and MAPK could be stimulated by TPA.

Several groups have found GnRH and its receptor expressed as part of an autocrine or paracrine regulation of human trophoblast and for modulation of placental functions during gestation[14–17,91–93] [72].

GnRH and its receptor were found to be expressed in many extra-pituitary tissues of different species, for example in human placental trophoblasts[15,94], human peripheral blood mononuclear cells[22], human ovary and granulosa cells[19,29], human and rat testis and ovary[95,96] or in different regions of the human brain[97]. The signal transduction of the GnRH receptor in extra-pituitary normal tissues has been only partly analyzed so far, but there are many signs that the mechanisms of GnRH action in extra-pituitary tissues are the same as those found in the pituitary[10,98,99].

HUMAN CANCERS

Expression of GnRH receptors in human cancers

In earlier studies it was shown that breast, ovarian, endometrial, pancreatic and prostatic cancers express specific binding sites for GnRH[1,2,4,100–104]. Although these GnRH binding sites had a molecular mass comparable with that of the pituitary GnRH receptor, their binding characteristics were of the low-affinity/high-capacity type[4,103–105]. Later it become evident that, in breast, ovarian, endometrial and prostate cancer cell lines, as well as in the respective biopsy samples, two types of GnRH binding site exist: one of low affinity and high capacity, the other of high affinity and low capacity. The latter is comparable to the pituitary GnRH receptor[4,103,104]. In 1992, the cloning, sequencing and expression of the human pituitary GnRH receptor was reported[26]. In the same publication, the authors reported the expression of mRNA for the human GnRH receptor in the breast cancer cell line MCF-7. These findings stimulated intensive research leading to the demonstration of GnRH receptor gene transcripts in ovarian and endometrial cancer cell lines and in about 80% of the respective primary tumors[104,106–108]. In ovarian and endometrial cancer specimens and cell lines expressing mRNA for the pituitary GnRH receptor, high-affinity/low-capacity binding sites were found to be closely related to the pituitary GnRH receptor[106–110]. Kakar and associates[28] demonstrated that the nucleotide sequence of GnRH receptors in human breast and ovarian tumors is identical to that found in the pituitary. Data available today suggest that about 50% of breast cancers[111] and approximately 80% of ovarian and endometrial cancers express high-affinity binding sites for GnRH. For prostate cancer, fewer findings have been published[103], but systematic investigations might lead to comparable results.

Expression of GnRH by human cancers

It has been known since the early 1980s that human milk as well as biopsy samples and cell lines of human breast cancers contain GnRH immunoreactivity[4,112]. In 1991, Harris and colleagues[12] reported the expression of the mRNA for GnRH in two human breast carcinoma cell lines. Recently, two groups independently demonstrated the expression of GnRH immunoreactivity, bioactivity and the mRNA for GnRH by cell lines and the majority of biopsy samples of ovarian and endometrial cancers[11,108,113]. Therefore, as breast, ovarian and endometrial cancers express GnRH and its receptor, it seems reasonable to speculate that in many of these tumors there is a local regulatory system based on GnRH. The same situation was found in prostate cancer cells[102].

Direct anti-tumor effects of GnRH analogues in human cancer cells

Direct inhibitory effects of GnRH agonists on the *in vitro* proliferation of human breast cancer cell lines were first demonstrated by Blankenstein and colleagues[114] and Miller and colleagues[115]. Subsequently, several groups provided evidence that the *in vitro* proliferation of a variety of human cancer cell lines could be inhibited by agonistic and/or antagonistic analogues of GnRH in a dose- and time-dependent manner[4,104,109,110,116,117]. In most cancer cells except the ovarian cancer cell line EFO-27, GnRH antagonists act as agonists, indicating that the dichotomy between GnRH agonists and antagonists does not exist in tumor cells[109,118]. Using human ovarian cancer cell line OV-1063 xenografted into nude mice, Yano and co-workers[119] demonstrated a significant inhibition of tumor growth by chronic treatment with the GnRH antagonist cetrorelix but not with the GnRH agonist triptorelin. As both GnRH analogues induced a comparable suppression of the pituitary–gonadal axis, the authors speculated that the anti-tumor effects of cetrorelix were exerted directly on GnRH receptors in tumors. The findings on direct anti-tumor effects of GnRH analogues in ovarian and endometrial cancer reported by others are completely or partly in agreement with the results described earlier here[104,120–122]. In contrast, other groups failed to detect direct anti-tumor effects of GnRH analogues in human ovarian and endometrial cancer cell lines or observed them only at extremely high GnRH analogue concentrations[123–125]. Some of these discrepancies might be explained by the fact that the majority of the cell lines used by these authors probably did not express high-affinity

GnRH receptors[104,126]. Alternatively, differences in culture or experimental conditions as well as in the types of GnRH analogues used might have been responsible for the observed variance. In the case of prostate cancer, several groups reported direct anti-proliferative effects of GnRH analogues *in vitro* and in animal *in vivo* models, which could be mediated through specific GnRH-binding sites[1,103,127–131] [22].

Molecular mechanisms mediating the direct anti-tumor effects of GnRH

In view of the apparent similarity of GnRH receptors in peripheral cancers to those in the pituitary, it seems reasonable to speculate that GnRH signal transduction pathways in tumors might also be comparable to those operating in pituitary gonadotrophs, such as phospholipase C and protein kinase C (see above). Early reports on GnRH signal transduction in rat mammary tumors, human breast cancer cell lines and membranes from ovarian cancer biopsies supported this concept[132–135]. Our group performed extensive studies in human ovarian (EFO-21, EFO-27) and endometrial (HEC-1A, Ishikawa) cancer cell lines. These cell lines express GnRH receptors, and their proliferation is inhibited by GnRH analogues[108–110]. Although we could clearly demonstrate the activation of phospholipase C, protein kinase C and adenylyl cyclase in the tumor cells by pharmacological stimuli, the GnRH agonist triptorelin, at concentrations that are clearly inhibitory to proliferation, had no effects on the activity of these signalling systems[136]. We found, however, that the mitogenic effect of growth factors (epidermal growth factor (EGF), insulin-like growth factor (IGF)) in these cell lines could be counteracted by triptorelin, indicating an interaction with the mitogenic signal transduction pathway[136] [23] (Figure 2). Comparable data were obtained by Moretti and colleagues[137] in the human prostatic cancer cell lines LNCaP and DU 145. These findings are in accordance with reports that GnRH analogues reduce expression of growth factor receptors and their mRNA[119,137,138] and/or growth factor-induced tyrosine kinase activity[134,136,137,139–143]. Growth factor-induced tyrosine phosphorylation is probably counteracted by GnRH analogues through activation of a phosphotyrosine phosphatase[136,137,139,140,142,143], which is probably coupled to the GnRH receptor through a Gi-protein in human reproductive tract tumors[144]. Imai and co-workers[144] speculated that the Gi-protein that couples the GnRH receptor to the effector may be responsible for the difference in response by the peripheral tumors and the anterior pituitary. The concept of an inhibition of mitogenic signal transduction by GnRH analogues in human cancer cells was further corroborated by our group. We demonstrated that EGF-induced activation of mitogen-activated protein kinase, an enzyme further downstream in the growth factor signalling cascade[145], was virtually blocked in ovarian and endometrial cancer cells treated with the GnRH agonist

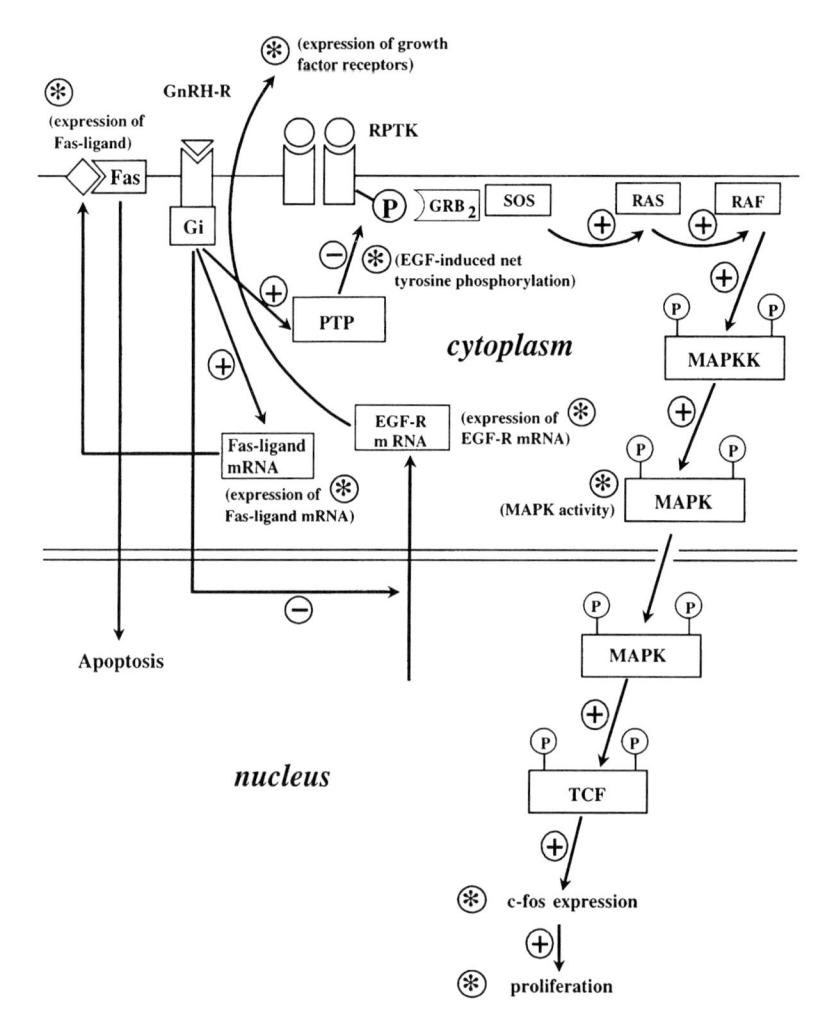

Figure 2 Hypothetical molecular mechanisms mediating the anti-proliferative effects of GnRH analogues in human cancer cells. Asterisk indicates mechanisms that have been shown to be involved in GnRH action. Modified according to Emons and colleagues[118] with supplements. For references and further details, see text

triptorelin[136]. By quantitative RT-PCR, our group showed that the EGF-induced expression of the immediate early gene c-*fos*, a mechanism still further downstream in mitogenic signalling, was completely abrogated in breast, ovarian and endometrial cancer cells by treatment with the GnRH agonist triptorelin as well as with the GnRH antagonist cetrorelix[146] [65]. The same effects were seen in the prostatic cancer cell line LNCaP by treatment with the GnRH agonist goserelin[137]. In prostatic cancer cells GnRH agonists inhibit proliferation by interfering with some of the cellular mechanisms mediating the stimulatory action of the EGF and the IGF system[137,147]. Sica and colleagues [77] found that GnRH is ineffective in regulating cell growth, when used alone in both hormone-sensitive and -insensitive prostate cancer cell lines. However, it counteracts the stimulatory effect of androgens on the proliferation of LNCaP cells, which respond to low dihydrotestosterone concentrations. GnRH has an inhibitory effect on the mitogenic action of EGF in androgen-unresponsive PC-3 cells. It counteracts the androgen-induced gene expression in LNCaP cells and the EGF-induced gene expression in PC-3 cells. GnRH seems to act as a negative growth factor [77]. Other possible molecular mechanisms that might be involved in the mediation of the anti-tumor effects of GnRH analogues have also been suggested[104]. The reasons for the differences in GnRH signal transduction in pituitary and peripheral cancers are still unclear. Experimentally induced mutations of the GnRH receptor have altered GnRH binding, G-protein–receptor interaction, or proper membrane incorporation[148–154], but in none of the analyzed breast, endometrial and ovarian cancer cell lines did we find any mutation in the coding region of the GnRH receptor gene. Therefore, the GnRH receptor itself cannot be responsible for the changed GnRH signal transduction pathway in cancer cells[155]. On the other hand, some normal and neoplastic human tissues were found to express differential splice variants of the GnRH receptor gene in a tissue-dependent manner (Kottler and colleagues, unpublished data). It is not yet clear whether these splice variants can be translated into active membrane receptors or not. However, in the tumor cell lines analyzed by us, no signs for alternative GnRH receptor splice variants were seen. Active mutations of the G-protein have been implicated in the pathogenesis of some human neoplasms including ovarian tumors[144,156]. It is possible that G-protein mutations or unknown subtypes are responsible for the GnRH signalling in tumors and therefore for its anti-proliferative actions. In addition, it has been postulated that GnRH agonist-induced inhibition of cell proliferation is based on the increasing intracellular concentrations of annexin V, an effect mediated by the activation of PKC[117][74,75].

GnRH analogues and apoptosis

Apoptosis is an evolutionarily conserved form of programmed cell death[157–160]. The cell surface receptor protein Fas triggers apoptosis in a variety of cell types when cross-linked with the Fas ligand[161]. Fas is a single-chain polypeptide with a single transmembrane domain[162]. GnRH-induced anti-proliferative action may be mediated by stimulating apoptotic cell death[121,163]. GnRH has recently been shown to increase Fas ligand expression within the plasma membrane[164], known to promote apoptotic cell death through attack on Fas-positive cells within tumors. GnRH analogues are able to induce Fas ligand production in GnRH receptor-positive ovarian and endometrial cancer cells[165,166]. GnRH stimulation can directly inhibit the growth of Fas-positive endometrial cancer cells through Fas ligand expression. Therefore, the Fas/Fas ligand system linked to GnRH receptor activation may be one of the candidates for mediation of the anti-proliferative action of GnRH analogues by increasing apoptotic cell death within the tumor[165,166].

The GnRH antagonist cetrorelix is able to enhance apoptosis in endometrial cancer cell lines[121]. Yano and co-workers [76] found that the extent of apoptosis induced by the GnRH antagonist cetrorelix is greater than that following treatment with the GnRH agonist buserelin.

SUMMARY AND FUTURE PERSPECTIVES

GnRH receptors in the human pituitary, human normal extra-pituitary tissues and human cancers seem to be similar; their signal transduction mechanisms, however, appear to be different. In the pituitary, the mechanisms of action of GnRH are well understood, although the picture is becoming more and more complex. Many differential cross-talks between different pathways might mediate the diverse effects of GnRH on gonadotropin synthesis and release as well as on GnRH receptor expression. In human cancers the mechanisms of action are completely different. The dichotomy between GnRH agonists and antagonists based on pituitary response may not be applicable to the GnRH system found in cancer cells. In addition, the GnRH signal transduction pathway that operates in normal tissues seems not to be essential in cancer cells. The most important features in GnRH signalling in tumors are the inhibitory interference with the mitogenic pathway resulting in antiproliferative actions and the possibility to induce apoptosis. Since mutations in the GnRH receptor have not been detected so far, other factors might be responsible for the different GnRH signal transduction pathway in cancer cells. It might be speculated that minor mutations of the G-protein to which GnRH receptors are coupled in tumor cells could be responsible for these phenomena. In addition, it is probable that the GnRH systems in cancer cells are not uniform and that differences exist even between individual cancer cell lines and their subclones. These issues ought to be solved by further research, which might open new therapeutic options.

REFERENCES

1. Schally AV. Hypothalamic hormones from neuroendocrinology to cancer therapy. *Anticancer Drugs* 1994;5:115–130
2. Stojilkovic SS, Catt KJ. Expression and signal transduction pathways of gonadotropin-releasing hormone receptors. *Rec Prog Horm Res* 1995;30:161–205

3. Stanislaus D, Pinter JH, Janovick JA, Conn PM. Mechanisms mediating multiple physiological responses to gonadotropin-releasing hormone. *Mol Cell Endocrinol* 1998;144:1–10
4. Emons G, Schally AV. The use of luteinizing hormone-releasing hormone agonists and antagonists in gynecological cancers. *Hum Reprod* 1994;9:1364–79
5. Albano C, Smitz J, Camus M, Riethmüller-Winzen H, Van Steirteghem A, Devroey P. Comparison of different doses of gonadotropin-releasing hormone antagonist cetrorelix during controlled ovarian hyperstimulation. *Fertil Steril* 1997;67:917–22
6. Behre HM, Klein B, Steinmeyer E, McGregor GP, Voigt K, Nieschlag E. Effective supression of luteinizing hormone and testosterone by single doses of the new gonadotropin-releasing hormone antagonist cetrorelix (SB-75) in normal men. *J Clin Endocrinol Metab* 1992;75:393–8
7. Schally AV, Comaru-Schally AM. Hypothalamic and other peptide hormones. In Holland JF, Frei E III, Bast RR Jr, Kufe DE, Morton DL, Weichselbaum RR, eds. *Cancer Medicine*, Vol. 4. Baltimore: Williams and Wilkins, 1997:1067–86
8. Imai A, Iida K, Tamaya T. Tight coupling of gonadotropin-releasing hormone receptor to stimulated phosphoinositide turnover and antigonadotropic action in granulosa cells. *Gynecol Obstet Invest* 1992;33:36–41
9. Leung PC, Steele GL. Intracellular signaling in the gonads. *Endocr Rev* 1992;13:476–98
10. Stojilkovic SS, Reinhart J, Catt KJ. GnRH receptors: structure and signal transduction pathways. *Endocr Rev* 1994;15:462–99
11. Ohno T, Imai A, Furui T, Takahashi K, Tamaya T. Presence of gonadotropin-releasing hormone and its messenger ribonucleic acid in human ovarian epithelial carcinoma. *Am J Obstet Gynecol* 1993;169:605–10
12. Harris N, Dutlow C, Eidne K, Dong KW, Roberts J, Millar RP. Gonadotropin-releasing hormone gene expression in MDA-MB-231 and ZR-75-1 breast carcinoma cell lines. *Cancer Res* 1991;51:2577–81
13. Hsueh AJ, Jones PB. Extrapituitary actions of gonadotropin-releasing hormone. *Endocr Rev* 1981;2:437–61
14. Merz WE, Erlewein C, Licht P, Harbarth P. The secretion of human chorionic gonadotropin as well as the α- and β-messenger ribonucleic acid levels are stimulated by exogenous gonadoliberin pulses applied to first trimester placenta in a superfusion culture system. *J Clin Endocrinol Metab* 1991;73:84–92
15. Lin LS, Roberts VJ, Yen SS. Expression of human gonadotropin-releasing hormone receptor gene in placenta and its functional relationship to human chorionic gonadotropin secretion. *J Clin Endocrinol Metab* 1995;80:580–5
16. Bramley TA, McPhie CA, Menzies GS. Human placental gonadotropin-releasing hormone (GnRH) binding sites: I. Characterization, properties and ligand specifity. *Placenta* 1992;13:555–81
17. Bramley TA, McPhie CA, Menzies GS. Human placental gonadotropin-releasing hormone (GnRH) binding sites: III. Changes in GnRH binding levels with stage of gestation. *Placenta* 1994;15:733–45
18. Fraser HM, Sellar RE, Illingworth PJ, Eidne KA. GnRH receptor mRNA expression by *in-situ* hybridization in the primate pituitary and ovary. *Mol Hum Reprod* 1996;2:117–21
19. Peng C, Fan NC, Ligier M, Väänänen J, Leung PCK. Expression and regulation of gonadotropin-releasing hormone (GnRH) and GnRH receptor messenger ribonucleic acids in human granulosa–luteal cells. *Endocrinology* 1994;135:1740–5

20. Minaretzis D, Jakubowski M, Mortola JF, Pavlou SN. Gonadotropin-releasing hormone receptor gene expression in human ovary and granulosa–lutein cells. *J Clin Endocrinol Metab* 1995;80:430–4
21. Chegini N, Rong H, Dou Q, Kipersztok C, Williams RS. Gonadotropin-releasing hormone (GnRH) and GnRH receptor gene expression in human myometrium and leiomyomata and the direct action of GnRH analogs on myometrial smooth muscle cells and interaction with ovarian steroids *in vitro*. *J Clin Endocrinol Metab* 1996;81:3215–21
22. Chen HF, Jeung EB, Stephenson M, Leung PC. Human peripheral blood mononuclear cells express gonadotropin-releasing hormone (GnRH), GnRH receptor, and interleukin-2 receptor gamma-chain messenger ribonucleic acids that are regulated by GnRH *in vitro*. *J Clin Endocrinol Metab* 1999;84:743–50
23. Ho HN, Chen HF, Chen SU, et al. Gonadotropin-releasing hormone (GnRH) agonist induces down-regulation of the CD3+CD25+ lymphocyte subpopulation in peripheral blood. *Am J Reprod Immunol* 1995;33:243–52
24. Standaert FE, Chew BP, De Avila D, Reeves JJ. Presence of luteinizing hormone-releasing hormone binding sites in cultured porcine lymphocytes. *Biol Reprod* 1992;46:997–1000
25. Tsutsumi M, Zhou W, Millar RP, et al. Cloning and functional expression of a mouse gonadotropin-releasing hormone receptor. *Mol Endocrinol* 1992;6:1163–9
26. Kakar SS, Musgrove LC, Devor DC, Sellers JC, Neill JD. Cloning, sequencing, and expression of human gonadotropin-releasing hormone (GnRH) receptor. *Biochem Biophys Res Commun* 1992;189:289–95
27. Chi L, Zhou W, Prikhozan A, et al. Cloning and characterization of the human gonadotropin-releasing hormone receptor. *Mol Cell Endocrinol* 1993;91:R1–6
28. Kakar SS, Grizzle WE, Neill JD. The nucleotide sequence of human GnRH receptors in breast and ovarian tumors are identical with that found in pituitary. *Mol Cell Endocrinol* 1994;106:145–9
29. Sealfon SC, Millar RP. Functional domains of the gonadotropin-releasing hormone receptor. *Cell Mol Neurobiol* 1995;15:25–42
30. Sealfon SC, Millar RP. The gonadotropin-releasing hormone receptor: structural determinations and regulatory control. *Hum Reprod Update* 1995;1:216–30
31. Campion CE, Turzillo AM, Clay CM. The gene encoding the ovine gonadotropin-releasing hormone (GnRH) receptor: cloning and initial characterization. *Gene* 1996;170:277–80
32. Neer EJ. Heterotrimeric G proteins: organizers of transmembrane signals. *Cell* 1995;80:249–57
33. Heldin CH. Dimerization of cell surface receptors in signal transduction. *Cell* 1995;80:213–23
34. Davidson JS, Wakefield IK, Millar RP. Absence of rapid desensitization of the mouse gonadotropin-releasing hormone receptor. *Biochem J* 1994;300:299–302
35. Hsieh K-P, Martin TFJ. Thyrotropin-releasing hormone and gonadotropin-releasing hormone receptors activate phospholipase C by coupling to the guanosine triphosphate-binding proteins Gq and G_{11}. *Mol Endocrinol* 1992;6:1673–81
36. Naor Z. Signal transduction mechanism of Ca^{2+} mobilizing hormones. The case of gonadotropin-releasing hormone. *Endocr Rev* 1990;11:326–53

37. Stojilkovic SS, Tomic M, Kukuljan M, Catt KJ. Control of calcium spiking frequency in pituitary gonadotrophs by a single-pool cytoplasmic oscillator. *Mol Pharmacol* 1994;45:1013–21
38. Andrews WV, Conn PM. Gonadotropin-releasing hormone stimulates mass changes in phosphoinositides and diacylglycerol accumulation in purified gonadotrope cell cultures. *Endocrinology* 1986;118:1148–58
39. Reinhart J, Mertz LM, Catt KJ. Molecular cloning and expression of cDNA encoding the murine gonadotropin-releasing hormone receptors. *J Biol Chem* 1992;267:21281–4
40. Hawes BE, Waters SB, Janovick JA, Bleasdale JE, Conn PM. Gonadotropin-releasing hormone-stimulated intracellular Ca^{2+} fluctuations and luteinizing hormone release can be uncoupled from inositol phosphate production. *Endocrinology* 1992;130:3475–83
41. Limor R, Schvartz I, Hazum E, Ayalon D, Naor Z. Effect of guanine nucleotides on phospholipase C activity in permeabilized pituitary cells: possible involvement of an inhibitory GTP-binding protein. *Biochem Biophys Res Commun* 1989;159:209–15
42. Perrin MH, Haas Y, Porter J, Rivier J, Vale WW. The gonadotropin-releasing hormone pituitary receptor interactions with a guanosine triphosphate-binding protein: differential effects of guanyl nucleotides on agonist and antagonist binding. *Endocrinology* 1989;124:798–804
43. Shah BH, Milligan G. The gonadotropin-releasing hormone receptor of αT3-1 pituitary cells regulates cellular levels of both of the phosphoinositidase C-linked G proteins $Gq\alpha$ and $G_{11}\alpha$ equally. *Mol Pharmacol* 1994;46:1–7
44. Stanislaus D, Janovick JA, Brothers S, Conn PM. Regulation of $G_{(q/11)}$alpha by the gonadotropin-releasing hormone receptor. *Mol Endocrinol* 1997;11:738–46
45. Cornea A, Janovick JA, Stanislaus D, Conn PM. Redistribution of $G_{(q/11)}$alpha in the pituitary gonadotrope in response to a gonadotropin-releasing hormone agonist. *Endocrinology* 1998;139:397–402
46. Naor Z, Azrad A, Limor R, Zakut H, Lotan M. Gonadotropin-releasing hormone activates a rapid Ca^{2+}-independent phosphodiester hydrolysis of polyphosphoinositides in pituitary gonadotrophs. *J Biol Chem* 1986;261:12506–12
47. Morgan RO, Chang JP, Catt KJ. Novel aspects of gonadotropin-releasing hormone action on inositol polyphosphate metabolism in cultured pituitary gonadotrophs. *J Biol Chem* 1987;262:1166–71
48. Horn F, Bilezikjian LM, Perrin MH, *et al.* Intracellular responses to gonadotropin-releasing hormone in a clonal cell line of gonadotrope lineage. *Mol Endocrinol* 1991;5:347–55
49. Naor Z. GnRH receptor signalling: cross-talk of Ca^{2+} and protein kinase C. *Eur J Endocrinol* 1997;136:123–7
50. Naor Z, Catt KJ. Mechanism of action of gonadotropin-releasing hormone-involvement of phospholipid turnover in luteinizing hormone release. *J Biol Chem* 1981;256:2226–9
51. Naor Z. Is arachidonic acid a second messenger in signal transduction? *Mol Cell Endocrinol* 1991;80:181–6
52. Ben-Menahem D, Shraga-Levine Z, Limor R, Naor Z. Arachidonic acid and lipoxygenase products stimulate gonadotropin α-subunit mRNA levels in pituitary αT3-1 cell line: role in gonadotropin-releasing hormone action. *Biochemistry* 1994;33:12795–9

53. Netiv E, Liscivitch M, Naor Z. Delayed activation of phospholipase D by gonadotropin-releasing hormone in a clonal pituitary gonadotrope cell line (αT3-1). *FEBS Lett* 1991;295:107–9
54. Zheng L, Stojilkovic SS, Hunyady L, Krsmanovic LZ, Catt KJ. Sequential activation of phospholipase C and phospholipase D in agonist-stimulated gonadotrophs. *Endocrinology* 1994;134:1446–54
55. Nishizuka Y. The molecular heterogeneity of protein kinase C and its implications for cellular regulation. *Nature (London)* 1988;334:661–5
56. Asoaka Y, Nakamura S, Yoshida K, Nishizuka Y. Protein kinase C, calcium and phospholipid degradation. *Trends Biochem Sci* 1992;17:414–16
57. Nishizuka Y. Intracellular signaling by hydrolysis of phospholipids and activation of protein kinase C. *Science* 1992;258:607–14
58. Garcia-Navarro S, Kalina M, Naor Z. Immunocytochemical localization of protein kinase C subtypes in anterior pituitary cells: colocalization in hormone-containing cells reveals heterogeneity. *Endocrinology* 1991;129:2780–6
59. Huang KP. The mechanism of protein kinase C. *Trends Neurosci* 1989;12:425–32
60. Grunicke HH, Überall F. Protein kinase C modulation. *Semin Cell Biol* 1992;3:351–60
61. Omura S, Iwai Y, Hirano A, et al. A new alkaloid AM-2282 of *Streptomyces* origin: taxonomy, fermentation, isolation and preliminary characterisation. *J Antibiot* 1977;30:275–81
62. Tamaoki T, Nakano H. Potent and specific inhibitors of protein kinase C of microbial origin. *Biotechnology* 1990;8:732–5
63. Kikkawa U, Ogita K, Go M, et al. Protein kinase C in transmembrane signaling. *Adv Second Messenger Phosphoprotein Res* 1988;21:67–74
64. Newton AC. Protein kinase C: structure, function and regulation. *J Biol Chem* 1995;270:28495–8
65. Naor Z, Shearman MS, Kishimoto A, Nishizuka Y. Calcium-independent activation of hypothalamic type I protein kinase C by *cis*-unsaturated fatty acids. *Mol Endocrinol* 1988;2:1043–8
66. Bell RM, Burns DJ. Lipid activation of protein kinase C. *J Biol Chem* 1991;266:4661–4
67. Ben-Menahem D, Naor Z. Regulation of gonadotropin mRNA levels in cultured rat pituitary cells by gonadotropin-releasing hormone (GnRH): role of Ca^{2+} and protein kinase C. *Biochemistry* 1994;33:3698–704
68. Ben-Menahem D, Shraga-Levine Z, Mellon PL, Naor Z. Mechanism of action of gonadotropin-releasing hormone upon gonadotropin α-subunit gene expression in αT3-1 cell line: role for Ca^{2+} and protein kinase C. *Biochem J* 1995;309:325–9
69. Naor Z, Harris D, Shacham S. Mechanism of GnRH receptor signaling: combinatorial cross-talk of Ca^{2+} and protein kinase C. *Front Neuroendocrinol* 1998;19:1–9
70. Shraga-Levine Z, Ben-Menahem D, Naor Z. Activation of protein kinase Cβ gene expression by gonadotropin-releasing hormone in αT3-1 cell line: role of Ca^{2+} and autoregulation by protein kinase C. *J Biol Chem* 1994;269:31028–33
71. Harris D, Reiss N, Naor Z. Differential activation of protein kinase C δ and ε gene expression by gonadotropin-releasing hormone in αT3-1 cells: autoregulation by protein kinase C. *J Biol Chem* 1997;272:13534–40
72. Seger R, Krebs EG. The MAPK signaling cascade. *FASEB J* 1995;9:726–35

73. Reiss N, Nur-Levi L, Shacham S, Harris D, Seger R, Naor Z. Gonadotropin-releasing hormone activation of mitogen-activated protein (MAP) kinase in pituitary αT3-1 cell line: differential roles of calcium and protein kinase C. *Endocrinology* 1997;138:1673–82

74. Lin X, Conn PM. Transcriptional activation of gonadotropin-releasing hormone (GnRH) receptor gene by GnRH: involvement of multiple signal transduction pathways. *Endocrinology* 1999;140:358–64

75. Dan-Cohen H, Sofer Y, Schwartzmann ML, Natarajan RD, Nadler JL, Naor Z. GnRH activates the lipoxygenase pathway in cultured pituitary cells: role in gonadotropin secretion and evidence for a novel autocrine/paracrine loop. *Biochemistry* 1992;31:5442–8

76. Eberhardt I, Kiesel L. Role of arachidonic acid and lipoxygenase products in the mechanism of gonadotropin secretion: an update. *Prostaglandins Leukot Essent Fatty Acids* 1992;47:239–46

77. Shraga-Levine Z, Ben-Menahem D, Naor Z. Arachidonic acid and lipoxygenase products stimulate protein kinase Cβ mRNA levels in pituitary αT3-1 cell line: role in gonadotropin-releasing hormone action. *Biochem J* 1996;316:667–70

78. Levi NL, Hanoch T, Benard O, *et al.* Stimulation of Jun N-terminal kinase (JNK) by gonadotropin-releasing hormone in pituitary αT3-1 cell line is mediated by protein kinase C, c.Src, and CDC-42. *Mol Endocrinol* 1998;12:815–24

79. Davis RJ. MAPKs: new JNK expands the group. *Trends Biochem Sci* 1994;19:470–3

80. Karin M. The regulation of AP-1 activity by mitogen-activated protein kinases. *J Biol Chem* 1995;270:16483–6

81. Naor Z, Shacham S, Harris D, Seger R, Reiss N. Signal transduction of the gonadotropin-releasing hormone (GnRH) receptor: cross talk of calcium, protein kinase C (PKC) and arachidonic acid. *Cell Mol Neurobiol* 1996;15:527–44

82. Ortmann O, Emons G, Knuppen R, Catt KJ. Inhibitory actions of keoxifene on luteinizing hormone secretion in pituitary gonadotrophs. *Endocrinology* 1988;123:962–8

83. Ortmann O, Wiese H, Knuppen R, Emons G. Acute facilitatory action of progesterone on gonadotropin secretion of perfused rat pituitary cells. *Acta Endocrinol* 1989;121:426–34

84. Ortmann O, Emons G, Knuppen R, Catt KJ. Inhibitory effects of the antiprogestin, RU 486, on progesterone actions and luteinizing hormone secretion in pituitary gonadotrophs. *J Steroid Biochem* 1989;32:291–7

85. Ortmann O, Sturm R, Knuppen R, Emons G. Weak estrogenic activity of phenol red in the pituitary gonadotroph: re-evaluation of estrogen and antiestrogen effects. *J Steroid Biochem* 1990;35:17–22

86. Ortmann O, Stojilkovic SS, Cesnjaj M, Emons G, Catt KJ. Modulation of cytoplasmic calcium signaling in rat pituitary gonadotrophs by estradiol and progesterone. *Endocrinology* 1992;131:1565–8

87. Ortmann O, Tilse B, Emons G. Modulatory actions of estradiol and progesterone on phorbol ester-induced LH secretion from cultured rat pituitary cells. *J Steroid Biochem Mol Biol* 1992;43:619–27

88. Ortmann O, Johannsen K, Knuppen R, Emons G. Acute effects of estradiol and progesterone on melittin- and gonadotropin-releasing hormone-induced LH secretion. *J Endocrinol* 1992;132:251–9

89. Emons G, Pahwa GS, Brack C, Sturm R, Oberheuser F, Knuppen R. Gonadotropin releasing hormone binding sites in human epithelial ovarian carcinomata. *Eur J Cancer Clin Oncol* 1989;25:215–21

90. Emons G, Nill J, Sturm R, Ortmann O. Effects of progesterone on gonadotropin-releasing hormone receptor concentration in cultured estrogen-primed female rat pituitary cells. *J Steroid Biochem Mol Biol* 1992;42:831–9

91. Kakar SS, Jennes L. Expression of gonadotropin-releasing hormone and gonadotropin-releasing hormone receptor mRNAs in various non-reproductive human tissues. *Cancer Lett* 1995;98:57–62

92. Bramley TA, Menzies GS. Measurement of luteal and placental gonadotropin-releasing hormone (GnRH) binding sites: role of inactivation of GnRH tracer. *Mol Hum Reprod* 1996;2:535–9

93. Takeuchi S, Futamura N, Minoura H, Toyoda N. Possible direct effect of gonadotropin-releasing hormone on human endometrium and decidua. *Life Sci* 1998;62:1187–94

94. Wolfahrt S, Kleine B, Rossmanith WG. Detection of gonadotropin-releasing hormone and its receptor mRNA in human placental trophoblasts using *in-situ* reverse transcription-polymerase chain reaction. *Mol Hum Reprod* 1998;4:999–1006

95. Botte MC, Chamagne AM, Carre MC, Counis R, Kottler ML. Fetal expression of GnRH and GnRH receptor genes in rat testis and ovary. *J Endocrinol* 1998;159:179–89

96. Bahk JK, Hyun JS, Chung SH, *et al.* Stage specific identification of the expression of GnRH mRNA and localization of the GnRH receptor in mature rat and adult human testis. *J Urol* 1995;154:1958–61

97. Jennes L, Eyigor O, Janovick JA, Conn PM. Brain gonadotropin-releasing homone receptors: localization and regulation. *Recent Prog Horm Res* 1997;52:475–91

98. Liscovitch M, Amsterdam A. Gonadotropin-releasing hormone activates phospholipase D in ovarian granulosa cells. Possible role in signal transduction. *J Biol Chem* 1989;264:11762–7

99. Anderson L, Hillier SG, Eidne KA, Miro F. GnRH-induced calcium mobilisation and inositol phosphate production in immature and mature rat ovarian granulosa cells. *J Endocrinol* 1996;149:449–56

100. Friess H, Buchler M, Kiesel L, Krüger M, Beger HG. LH-RH receptors in the human pancreas. Basis for antihormonal treatment in ductal carcinoma of the pancreas. *Int J Pancreaticol* 1991;10:151–9

101. Baumann KH, Kiesel L, Kaufmann M, Bastert G, Runnebaum B. Characterization of binding sites for a GnRH-agonist (buserelin) in human breast cancer biopsies and their distribution in relation to tumor parameters. *Breast Cancer Res Treat* 1993;25:37–46

102. Dondi D, Limonta P, Moretti RM, Marelli MM, Garattini E, Motta M. Antiproliferative effects of luteinizing hormone-releasing hormone (LHRH) agonists on human androgen-independent prostate cancer cell line DU 145: evidence for an autocrine-inhibitory LHRH loop. *Cancer Res* 1994;54:4091–5

103. Loop SM, Gorder CA, Lewis SM, Saiers JH, Drivdahl RH, Ostenson RC. Growth inhibition of human prostatic cancer cells by an agonist of gonadotropin-releasing hormone. *Prostate* 1995;26:179–88

104. Emons G, Ortmann O, Schulz KD. GnRH analogues in ovarian, breast and endometrial cancers. In Lunenfeld B, Insler V, eds. *GnRH Analogues. The State of the Art 1996.* Carnforth, UK: Parthenon Publishing, 1996:95–120

105. Fekete M, Redding TW, Comaru-Schally AM, *et al.* Receptors for luteinizing hormone-releasing hormone, somatostatin, prolactin and epidermal growth factor in rat and human prostatic cancers and in benign prostatic hyperplasia. *Prostate* 1989;14:191–208

106. Imai A, Ohno T, Iida K, Fuseya T, Furui T, Tamaya T. Gonadotropin-releasing hormone receptors in gynecological tumors. *Cancer* 1994;74:2555–61

107. Imai A, Ohno T, Iida K, Fuseya T, Furui T, Tamaya T. Presence of gonadotropin-releasing hormone receptor and its messenger ribonucleic acid in endometrial carcinoma and endometrium. *Gynecol Oncol* 1994;55:114–18

108. Irmer G, Bürger C, Müller R, et al. Expression of the messenger RNAs for luteinizing hormone-releasing hormone (LHRH) and its receptor in human ovarian epithelial carcinoma. *Cancer Res* 1995;55:817–22

109. Emons G, Ortmann O, Becker M, et al. High affinity binding and direct antiproliferative effects of LHRH analogues in human ovarian cancer cell lines. *Cancer Res* 1993;54:5439–46

110. Emons G, Schröder B, Ortmann O, Westphalen S, Schulz KD, Schally AV. High affinity binding and direct antiproliferative effects of luteinizing hormone-releasing hormone analogs in human endometrial cancer cell lines. *J Clin Endocrinol Metab* 1993;77:1458–64

111. Fekete M, Wittliff JL, Schally AV. Characteristics and distribution of receptors for [D-Trp^6]-luteinizing hormone-releasing hormone, somatostatin, epidermal growth factor and sex steroids in 500 biopsy samples of human breast cancer. *J Clin Lab Anal* 1989;3:137–47

112. Kiesel L. Molecular mechanisms of gonadotropin-releasing hormone-stimulated gonadotropin secretion. *Hum Reprod* 1994;8(Suppl 2):23–8

113. Irmer G, Bürger C, Ortmann O, Schulz KD, Emons G. Expression of luteinizing hormone-releasing hormone and its mRNA in human endometrial cancer cell lines. *J Clin Endocrinol Metab* 1994;79:916–19

114. Blankenstein MA, Henkelman MS, Klijn JMG. Direct inhibitory effect of a luteinizing hormone-releasing hormone agonist on MCF-7 human breast cancer cells. *Eur J Cancer Clin Oncol* 1985;21:1493–9

115. Miller WR, Scott WN, Morris R, Fraser HM, Sharpe RM. Growth of human breast cancer cells inhibited by luteinizing hormone-releasing hormone agonist. *Nature (London)* 1985;313:231–3

116. Yano T, Pinski J, Radulovic S, Schally AV. Inhibition of human epithelial ovarian cancer cell growth *in vitro* by agonistic and antagonistic analogues of luteinizing hormone-releasing hormone. *Proc Natl Acad Sci USA* 1994;91:1701–4

117. Shibata S, Sato H, Ota H, Karube A, Takahashi O, Tanaka T. Involvement of annexin V in antiproliferative effects of gonadotropin-releasing hormone agonists on human endometrial cancer cell line. *Gynecol Oncol* 1997;66:217–21

118. Emons G, Ortmann O, Schulz KD, Schally AV. Growth-inhibitory actions of analogues of luteinizing hormone releasing hormone on tumor cells. *Trends Endocrinol Metab* 1997;8:355–62

119. Yano T, Pinski J, Halmos G, Szepeshazi K, Schally AV. Inhibition of growth of OV-1063 human epithelial ovarian cancer xenografts in nude mice by treatment with luteinizing hormone-releasing hormone antagonist SB-75. *Proc Natl Acad Sci USA* 1994;91:7090–4

120. Thompson MA, Adelson MD, Kaufman LM. Lupron retards proliferation of ovarian tumor cells cultured in serum-free medium. *J Clin Endocrinol Metab* 1991;72:1036–41

121. Kleinman D, Douvdevani A, Schally AV, Levy J, Sharoni Y. Direct growth inhibition of human endometrial cancer cells by the gonadotropin-releasing hormone antagonist SB-75: role of apoptosis. *Am J Obstet Gynecol* 1994;170:96–102

122. Pályi I, Vincze B, Kálnay A, et al. Effect of gonadotropin releasing hormone analogs and their conjugates on gonadotropin-releasing hormone receptor-positive human cancer cell lines. *Cancer Detect Prev* 1996;20:146–52

123. Connor JP, Buller RE, Conn PM. Effect of GnRH analogs on six ovarian cancer cell lines in culture. *Gynecol Oncol* 1994;54:3215–21

124. Manetta A, Gamboa-Vujicic L, Paredes P, et al. Inhibition of growth of human ovarian cancer in nude mice by luteinizing hormone-releasing hormone antagonist cetrorelix (SB-75). *Fertil Steril* 1995;63:282–7

125. Chatzaki E, Bax CMR, Eidne KA, Anderson L, Grudzinskas JG, Gallagher CJ. The expression of gonadotropin-releasing hormone and its receptor in endometrial cancer and its relevance as an autocrine growth factor. *Cancer Res* 1996;56:2055–65

126. Emons G, Ortmann O, Irmer G, Müller V, Schulz KD, Schally AV. Treatment of ovarian cancer with LHRH antagonists. In Filicori M, Flamigni C, eds. *Treatment with GnRH Analogs: Controversies and Perspectives*. Carnforth, UK: Parthenon Publishing, 1996: 165–72

127. Motta M, Dondi D, Moretti M, et al. Role of growth factors, steroid and peptide hormones in the regulation of human prostatic tumor growth. *J Steroid Biochem Mol Biol* 1996;56:107–11

128. Jungwirth A, Galvan G, Pinski J, et al. Luteinizing hormone releasing hormone antagonist Cetrorelix (SB-75) and bombesin antagonist RC-3940-II inhibit the growth of androgen-independent PC-3 prostate cancer in nude mice. *Prostate* 1997;32:164–72

129. Jungwirth A, Pinski J, Galvan G, et al. Inhibition of growth of androgen-independent DU-145 prostate cancer *in vivo* by luteinizing hormone-releasing hormone antagonist cetrorelix and bombesin antagonists RC-3940-II and RC-3950-II. *Eur J Cancer* 1997;33: 1141–8

130. Montagnani-Marelli M, Moretti RM, Dondi D, Limonta P, Motta M. Effects of LHRH agonists on the growth of human prostatic tumor cells: '*in vitro*' and '*in vivo*' studies. *Arch Ital Urol Androl* 1997;69:257–63

131. Qayum A, Gullick W, Clayton RC, Sikora K, Waxman J. The effects of gonadotropin-releasing hormone analogues in prostate cancer are mediated through specific tumor receptors. *Br J Cancer* 1990;62:96–9

132. Levy J, Segal T, Wiznitzner A, Insler V, Sharoni Y. Molecular mechanisms of GnRH action on mammary tumors and uterine leiomyomata. In Vickery BH, Lunenfeld B, eds. *GnRH Analogues in Cancer and Human Reproduction*, Vol. 1. Dordrecht: Kluwer, 1989: 127–35

133. Segal-Abramson T, Giot J, Levy J, Sharoni Y. Guanine nucleotide modulations of high affinity gonadotropin-releasing hormone receptors in rat mammary tumors. *Mol Cell Endocrinol* 1992;85:105–16

134. Kéri G, Balogh A, Szöke B, Téplan J, Csika O. Gonadotropin-releasing hormone analogues inhibit cell proliferation and activate signal transduction pathways in MDA-MB-231 human breast cancer cell lines. *Tumor Biol* 1991;12:61–7

135. Imai A, Ohno T, Furui T, Takahashi K, Matsuda T, Tamaya T. Gonadotropin-releasing hormone stimulates phospholipase C but not protein phosphorylation/dephosphorylation in plasma membrane from human epithelial ovarian cancer. *Int J Gynecol Cancer* 1993;3: 311–17

136. Emons G, Müller V, Ortmann O, et al. Luteinizing hormone-releasing hormone agonist triptorelin antagonizes signal transduction and mitogenic activity of epidermal growth factor in human ovarian and endometrial cancer cell lines. *Int J Oncol* 1996;9:1129–37
137. Moretti RM, Montagnani-Marelli M, Dondi D, et al. Luteinizing hormone-releasing hormone agonists interfere with the stimulatory actions of epidermal growth factor in human prostatic cancer cell lines, LNCaP and DU 145. *J Clin Endocrinol Metab* 1996;81:3930–7
138. Shirahige Y, Cook C, Pinski J, Halmos G, Nair R, Schally AV. Treatment with luteinizing hormone-releasing hormone antagonist SB-75 decreases levels of epidermal growth factor receptor and its mRNA in OV-1063 human epithelial ovarian cancer xenografts in nude mice. *Int J Oncol* 1994;5:1031–5
139. Lee MT, Liebow C, Kramer AR, Schally AV. Effects of epidermal growth factor and analogues of luteinizing hormone-releasing hormone and somatostatin on phosphorylation of tyrosine residues of specific substrates in various tumors. *Proc Natl Acad Sci USA* 1991;88:1656–60
140. Liebow C, Lee MT, Kramer AR, Schally AV. Regulation of luteinizing hormone-releasing hormone receptor binding by heterologous receptor-stimulated tyrosine phosphorylation. *Proc Natl Acad Sci USA* 1991;88:2244–8
141. Hershkovitz E, Marbach M, Bosin M, et al. Luteinizing hormone-releasing hormone antagonists interfere with autocrine and paracrine growth stimulation of MCF-7 mammary cancer cells by insulin like growth factors. *J Clin Endocrinol Metab* 1993;77:963–8
142. Imai A, Takagi H, Furui T, Horibe S, Fuseya T, Tamaya T. Evidence for coupling of phosphotyrosine phosphatase to gonadotropin-releasing hormone receptor in ovarian carcinoma membrane. *Cancer* 1996;77:132–7
143. Furui T, Imai A, Takagi H, Horibe S, Fuseya T, Tamaya T. Phosphotyrosine phosphatase activity in membranes from endometrial carcinoma. *Oncol Rep* 1995;2:1055–7
144. Imai A, Takagi H, Horibe S, Fuseya T, Tamaya T. Coupling of gonadotropin releasing hormone receptor to Gi protein in human reproductive tract tumors. *J Clin Endocrinol Metab* 1996;81:3249–53
145. Hunter T. Protein kinases and phosphatases: the yin and yang of protein phosphorylation and signaling. *Cell* 1995;80:225–36
146. Gründker C, Völker P, Schulz KD, Emons G. GnRH agonists and antagonists inhibit the EGF-induced c-fos expression in endometrial, ovarian and breast cancer cell lines. *Exp Clin Endocrinol Diabetes* 1999;107(Suppl 1):81
147. Montagnani-Marelli M, Moretti RM, Dondi D, Motta M, Limonta P. Luteinizing hormone-releasing hormone agonists interfere with mitogenic activity of the insulin-like growth factor system in androgen-independent prostate cancer cells. *Endocrinology* 1999;140:329–34
148. Cook JV, Faccenda E, Anderson L, Couper GG, Eidne KA, Taylor PL. Effects of Asn87 and Asp318 mutations on ligand binding and signal transduction in the rat GnRH receptor. *J Endocrinol* 1993;139:R1–4
149. Zhou W, Flanagan C, Ballesteros JA, et al. A reciprocal mutation supports helix 2 and helix 7 proximity in the gonadotropin-releasing hormone receptor. *Mol Pharmacol* 1994;45:165–70

150. Davidson JS, Flanagan CA, Zhou W, et al. Identification of *N*-glycosylation sites in the gonadotropin-releasing homone receptor: role in receptor expression but not ligand binding. *Mol Cell Endocrinol* 1995;107:241–5
151. Fan NC, Peng C, Krisinger J, Leung PC. The human gonadotropin-releasing hormone receptor gene: complete structure including multiple promotors, transcription initiation sites, and polyadenylation signals. *Mol Cell Endocrinol* 1995;107:R1–8
152. Clapham DE. Direct G-protein activation of ion channels? *Annu Rev Neurosci* 1994;17:441–64
153. Sharif M, Sasakawa N, Hanley MR. Malignant transformation by G protein-coupled hormone receptors. *Mol Cell Endocrinol* 1994;100:115–19
154. Strader CD, Fong TM, Tota MR, Underwood D, Dixon RA. Structure and function of G protein-coupled receptors. *Annu Rev Biochem* 1994;63:101–32
155. Gründker C, Völker P, Herrmann L, Schulz KD, Emons G. GnRH inhibits the EGF-induced c-fos expression in endometrial and ovarian cancer. *Arch Gynecol Obstet* 1998;261(Suppl 1):146
156. Raymond JR. Multiple mechanisms of receptor-G protein signaling specificity. *Am J Physiol* 1995;269:F141–58
157. Hetts SW. To die or not to die: an overview of apoptosis and its role in disease. *J Am Med Assoc* 1998;279:300–7
158. Kerr JF, Gobe GC, Winterford CM, Harmon BV. Anatomical methods in cell death. *Methods Cell Biol* 1994;46:1–27
159. Nagata S. Apoptosis by death factor. *Cell* 1997;88:355–65
160. Thompson CB. Apoptosis in the pathogenesis and treatment of disease. *Science* 1995;267:1456–62
161. Nagata S, Golstein P. The Fas death factor. *Science* 1995;267:1449–1456
162. Itoh N, Yonehara S, Ishii A, et al. The polypeptide encoded by the cDNA for human cell surface antigen Fas can mediate apoptosis. *Cell* 1991;66:233–43
163. Schwartzman RA, Cidlowski JA. Apoptosis: the biochemistry and molecular biology of programmed cell death. *Endocr Rev* 1993;14:133–51
164. Imai A, Horibe S, Takagi A, Ohno T, Tamaya T. Frequent expression of Fas in gonadotropin-releasing hormone receptor-bearing tumors. *Eur J Obstet Gynecol Reprod Biol* 1997;74:73–8
165. Imai A, Takagi A, Horibe S, Takagi H, Tamaya T. Evidence for tight coupling of gonadotropin-releasing hormone receptor to stimulate Fas ligand expression in reproductive tumors: possible mechanism for hormonal control of apoptotic cell death. *J Clin Endocrinol Metab* 1998;83:127–431
166. Imai A, Takagi A, Horibe S, Takagi H, Tamaya T. Fas and Fas-ligand system may mediate antiproliferative activity of gonadotropin-releasing hormone receptor in endometrial cancer cells. *Int J Oncol* 1998;13:97–100

BIBLIOGRAPHY

Abstracts of relevant papers presented at the 5th International Symposium on GnRH Analogues in Cancer and Human Reproduction

19. GnRH signaling in the pituitary: from receptor to nucleus. Z. Naor, R. Seger, Israel
20. GnRH receptor and potential action in human ovary. P.C.K. Leung, Canada
21. GnRH-signaling in uterine myoma and in the intact mammary gland. Y. Koch, L.N. Levi, J. Adler, Israel
22. Direct antiproliferative effect of LHRH agonists on human prostatic tumor cells: possible mechanism of action. M. Motta, Italy
23. GnRH-signal transduction in breast, ovarian and endometrial cancers. G. Emons, C. Gründker, P. Völker, Germany
64. First results of the GnRH-antagonist cetrorelix in patients with ovarian cancer. G. Emons, S. Westphalen, K.-D. Schulz, *et al.*, Germany
65. GnRH reduces endometrial, ovarian and breast cancer cell proliferation via inhibition of growth factor-induced mitogenic signal transduction. C. Gründker, P. Völker, K.-D. Schulz, G. Emons, Germany
67. Pharmacodynamic effects of single doses of teverelix in healthy men. K. Erb, P. Ruus, A. Schüler, R. Deghenghi, R. Hermann, Germany
68. Pharmacokinetic characteristics of ganirelix (Orgalutran™) and its suppressive effect on the pituitary–gonadal axis. J. Oberjé, B. Mannaerts, J. Huisman, H.J. Kleijn, The Netherlands
72. GnRH and GnRH receptor in human trophoblasts: a model for autocrine regulation? B. Kleine, S. Wolfahrt, H. Jarry, W.G. Rossmanith, Germany
74. Involvement of annexin V in antiproliferative effect of GnRH agonists on cultured human uterine leiomyoma cells. H. Yamamoto, S. Shibata, M. Murata, *et al.*, Japan
75. Effects of GnRH agonists on the cell growth of ovarian and endometrial carcinoma cell lines. N. Ohyama, J. Xin Qiang, S. Shibata, *et al.*, Japan
76. Inhibition of human epithelial ovarian cancer cell growth *in vivo* and *in vitro* by GnRH analogues. T. Yano, N. Yano, H. Matsumi, H. Jimbo, Y. Taketani, Japan
77. Leuprorelin acetate regulates cell growth and PSA gene expression in prostatic cancer cells. G. Sica, F. Iacopino, G. Schinzari, D. Settesoldi, G. Zelano, Italy

2
GnRH analogues towards the next millennium

J. Rivier

My thanks go to Professor Lunenfeld and the Organizing Committee for the invitation to serve as rapporteur for the Session entitled 'GnRH Analogues Towards the Next Millennium' and related presentations. I was given this same opportunity 6 years ago and think that a short summary of the issues discussed at that time could serve as a good introduction. At that time, gonadotropin releasing hormone (GnRH) antagonists were labelled 'drugs of the future' with some of us very doubtful of their chances; now, we are all convinced that they will be drugs in the very near future. This is a major step forward that resulted from years of effort directed at finding adequate formulations of GnRH antagonists with distinct physicochemical properties. Other issues of concern were related to the commercial viability of GnRH antagonists that depended on their lack of histamine-releasing activity and their ability to be formulated for once-a-month administration at a competitive cost. I am happy to report that the reason these issues were not discussed at this meeting is that using GnRH antagonists for all indications benefiting from inhibition of gonadotropins is now conceptually accepted and that many technical difficulties associated with the implementation of their use have been solved.

Still of some concern is the ability of some of the GnRH antagonists to form gels or the inability of some of the long-lasting formulations to deliver enough of the antagonist for sustained inhibition of gonadal functions after a single administration without a 'loading' phase. I will address these concerns later as I summarize the contributions of Broqua and colleagues, describing preclinical data of a newcomer in the field (FE200486) [18], Boutignon and colleagues, describing the effect of a single injection of Antarelix® depot (teverelix) in dogs [78], Hutchison and colleagues, describing clinical investigations with azaline B [17], Molineaux and colleagues, describing early clinical uses of abarelix depot [16] and myself and my colleagues, describing a new tool for the design of non-peptide GnRH [15]. Whole

Table 1 Structures of GnRH antagonists

Name	Structure	Reference
Antarelix	Ac-DNal-DCpa-DPal-Ser-Tyr-DHci-Leu-ILys-Pro-DAla-NH$_2$	1
Azaline B	Ac-DNal-DCpa-DPal-Ser-Aph(Atz)-DAph(Atz)-Leu-ILys-Pro-DAla-NH$_2$	2
Abarelix	Ac-DNal-DCpa-DPal-Ser-N-MeTyr-DAsn-Leu-ILys-Pro-DAla-NH$_2$	3
Ganirelix	Ac-DNal-DCpa-DPal-Ser-Tyr-DHArg(Et$_2$)-Leu-HArg(Et$_2$)-Pro-DAla-NH$_2$	4
Cetrorelix	Ac-DNal-DCpa-DPal-Ser-Tyr-DCit-Leu-Arg-Pro-DAla-NH$_2$	5
FE200486	not available	

sessions were dedicated to the discussion of the properties of ganirelix depot and cetrorelix pamoate, which will not be discussed here.

The structures of GnRH antagonists described at this meeting (when available) are shown in Table 1.

PRESENTATION BY BROQUA AND COLLEAGUES [18]

In his first slides, Dr Broqua presented data in the castrated male rat comparing dose–response curves of abarelix, ganirelix, cetrorelix, azaline B and FE200486, where the volume of subcutaneous injection in 5% mannitol was kept constant at 0.4 ml/kg. Ganirelix and abarelix, at doses of up to 200 µg/kg showed rapid onset of inhibition of luteinizing hormone (LH) that lasted less than 24 h. At the dose of 200 µg/kg, cetrorelix-induced inhibition of LH lasted a little less than 3 days. By comparison, azaline B inhibited LH for 4–5 days and FE200486 inhibited LH for 5–6 days. Ganirelix, abarelix and cetrorelix did not show a clear dose-dependent increase in duration of action with increasing doses and concentrations (12.5, 50 and 200 µg/kg). However, azaline B and FE200486 produced a remarkable dose-dependent increase in duration of action, suggesting that further increases in the dose would allow long-term suppression of gonadotropins. Indeed, increasing the dose and concentration of azaline B and FE200486 ten-fold (2 m/kg in 20 µl 5% mannitol, subcutaneously) yielded complete inhibition of LH for 14 and 41 days, respectively. These results with azaline B whereby a ten-fold increase in dose resulted in a three-fold increase in duration of action were unexpected and disappointing. This was in fact addressed by Dr Hutchison [17], who showed that

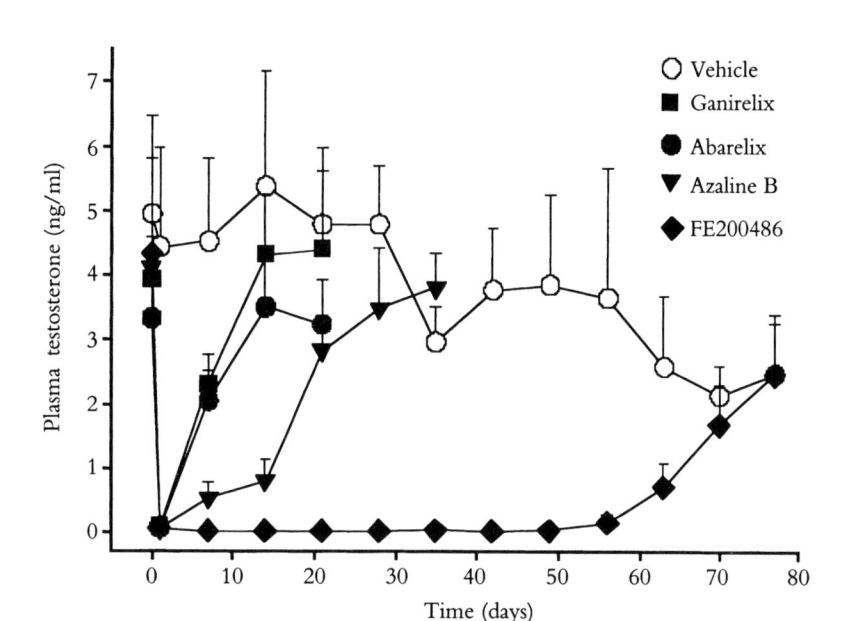

Figure 1 Long-term suppression of plasma testosterone in the intact rat by a single injection of FE200486 at 2 mg/kg (subcutaneously, 5% mannitol, 20 µl per animal)

increasing the concentration of azaline B beyond a certain point dramatically affected bioavailability in humans. This was explained by the tendency of azaline B to form gels beyond a certain concentration, gels that will not effectively reach the circulation at a rate that is sufficient to maintain LH inhibition. On the other hand, the same increase in dose of FE200486 resulted in a seven-fold increase in duration of action.

The question remained as to whether the profound and long-lasting inhibition of LH seen using a single injection of FE200486 would translate into similar inhibition of testosterone in the normal rat. Seven days after administration of ganirelix and abarelix (200 µg/kg in 20 µl 5% mannitol, subcutaneously) in intact rats, plasma testosterone had almost returned to baseline levels, demonstrating the need for these compounds to be formulated as slow-release preparations. Indeed, abarelix depot at 3 mg/kg produced suppression of testosterone for 28 days [16]. Under the same conditions, azaline B, which suppressed LH in castrated male rats for 2 weeks, also decreased testosterone levels in the intact rat for 2 weeks, although some rats had already escaped from castrate levels by day 7. By comparison, FE200486, at the same dose (Figure 1), maintained testosterone at castrate levels for 49 days, with one animal out of eight escaping by day 56. Testosterone levels then gradually increased to return to baseline levels at day 77. As expected, rats sacrificed at day 45 had considerably reduced weights of prostate, seminal vesicles and testes. Of all analogues tested, FE200486 was the least potent at releasing histamine from rat peritoneal mast cells and had the lowest cutaneous anaphylactoid activity.

PRESENTATION BY BOUTIGNON AND COLLEAGUES [78]

Teverelix (Antarelix®) shares its first five and last two amino acids with ganirelix and cetrorelix. It is different from cetrorelix in that it has a homocitrulline at position 6 instead of citrulline, and an isopropyllysine at position 8 instead of arginine, which is known to promote histamine-releasing activity. It is therefore less potent than cetrorelix at releasing histamine and otherwise very similar in most of its other properties[6]. A breakthrough in drug delivery was the discovery of a method to formulate teverelix as the soluble acetate salt using a proprietary process to give solvent-free biodegradable microgranules. This formulation (20 mg teverelix microcapsules suspended in an appropriate medium) was administered to male beagle dogs ($n = 6$; 13–15 kg). Testosterone levels were determined by an adapted commercial radio-immunoassay (RIA; Maia, Biodata, Biochem Immunosystems) and teverelix levels were determined by a validated RIA. The formulations were analyzed *in vitro* using a flow-through system (Erweka) equilibrated in Ringer solution with a flow rate of 0.5 ml/min. The released peptide was assayed using a reverse phase high-performance liquid chromatography (HPLC) method.

As presented in Figure 2, the dogs had undetectable testosterone levels for 25 days, after which time inhibition persisted at average levels below 0.5 ng/ml until day 48. After this time until day 80, the confidence limits were not significantly different from 0.5 ng/ml, the upper limit that the authors set as castrated levels. The pharmacokinetic profile showed a constant release that maintained levels of the drug, following an initial burst, at about 2–3 ng/ml until day 50. These pharmacokinetic data are similar to those obtained *in vitro*. Cumulative release over 45 days (60% of total), after a 24-h burst of about 15%, was followed by a zero-order release (no plateau) throughout the study (Figure 3).

The testosterone inhibition data presented in Figure 2 show profound inhibition of testosterone in the dog until day 25, at which time the concentration of the antagonist was around 5 ng/ml. Inhibition was then sustained for an additional 55 days during which period the concentration of Antarelix remained around 2 ng/ml at least until day 50. These results suggest that the minimal active concentration of Antarelix in the dog is likely to be less than 2 ng/ml.

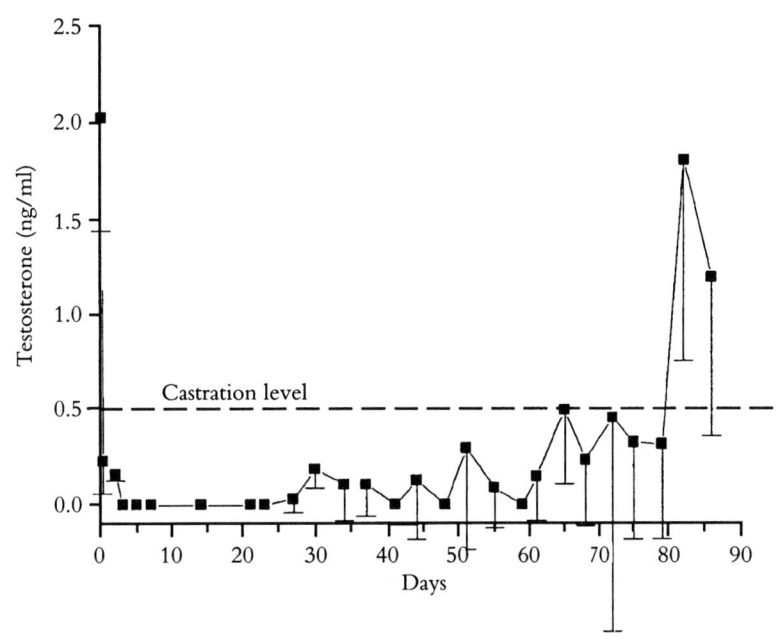

Figure 2 Long-term suppression of plasma testosterone in the intact beagle dog by a single injection (20 mg) of teverelix microgranules (subcutaneously in proprietary medium)

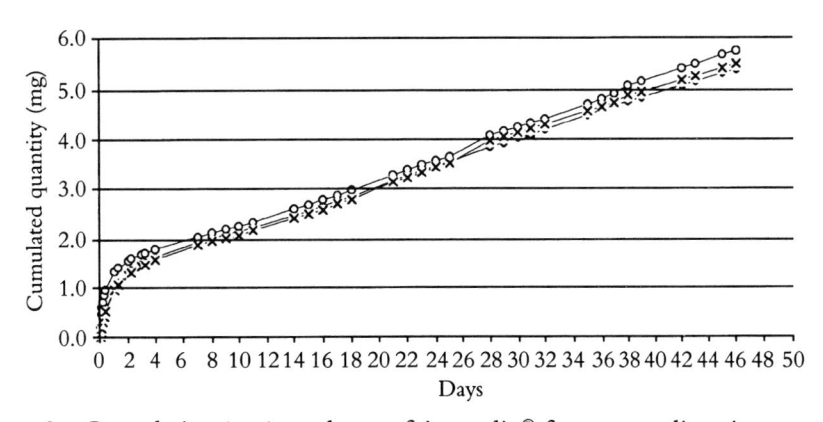

Figure 3 Cumulative *in vitro* release of Antarelix® from teverelix microgranules

PRESENTATION BY MOLINEAUX AND COLLEAGUES [16]

In the structure of abarelix we find the classical N-terminal tetrapeptide found in all other structures and an N-Me-tyrosine at position 5 that had been shown to increase solubility dramatically by preventing β-sheet formation around the turn defined by residues 5–8[7]. The introduction of a D-asparagine at position 6 (in lieu of bulky hydrophobic aromatic residues or citrulline/ homocitrulline) is original, while amino acids at positions 7–10 are those optimized for the blunting of histamine-releasing properties (ILys[8]) and stability against enzyme degradation (DAla[10]). As a result of these modifications, abarelix (PPI-149) is a potent competitive GnRH antagonist with high water solubility and low histamine-releasing activity but short duration of action. What was reported was a novel sustained-release formulation of abarelix (referred to as abarelix-depot developed at PRAECIS) and its pharmacological and pharmacokinetic behavior in mice, rats, dogs and monkeys prior to initiation of clinical studies. Results in dogs (single and multiple injections) and rats (single injection) are shown in Figures 4 and 5.

Abarelix depot was administered to animals as single or multiple intramuscular or subcutaneous doses. The efficacy of abarelix was determined by measurement of the plasma concentration of testosterone throughout the studies. Plasma levels of abarelix were determined by RIA using a sensitive and specific polyclonal antibody. Alternatively, radioactivity was determined in plasma, urine, feces and in 35 different tissues following administration of [^{14}C]abarelix depot in rats in order to establish the absorption, distribution and elimination of abarelix. Gonadal suppression was confirmed by histological demonstration of organ regression.

The minimal acceptable profile (that was met) of a depot formulation of abarelix included rapid suppression of plasma testosterone/estrogen following intramuscular or subcutaneous administration, maintenance of suppression for more than 28 days, reversibility of androgen/estrogen ablation following discontinuation, and safety and ease of manufacture. Indeed, administration of abarelix depot to dogs and rats as a single intramuscular or subcutaneous injection resulted in rapid, sustained suppression of plasma testosterone lasting more than 28 days. The plasma concentration of abarelix was shown to rise over the first 3–4 days after intramuscular or subcutaneous administration and to decline exponentially over the next month.

Doses of 1.2 to 3 mg/kg abarelix depot given to dogs at 28-day intervals for 1 year resulted in sustained, castrate levels of plasma testosterone. Dogs recovered normal plasma testosterone levels 4–6 weeks after discontinuation of therapy; the testicular histology was indistinguishable from that of normal dogs after 3 months.

The plasma time–concentration profile of [^{14}C]abarelix depot in rats was consistent with a 'flip/flop' pharmacokinetic mechanism wherein the elimination rate constant (K_e) is much greater than the absorption rate constant (K_a). There was no significant accumulation of radioactivity in any tissue. Fecal (70%) and urinary (30%) excretion were the major pathways of elimination of [^{14}C]abarelix. The

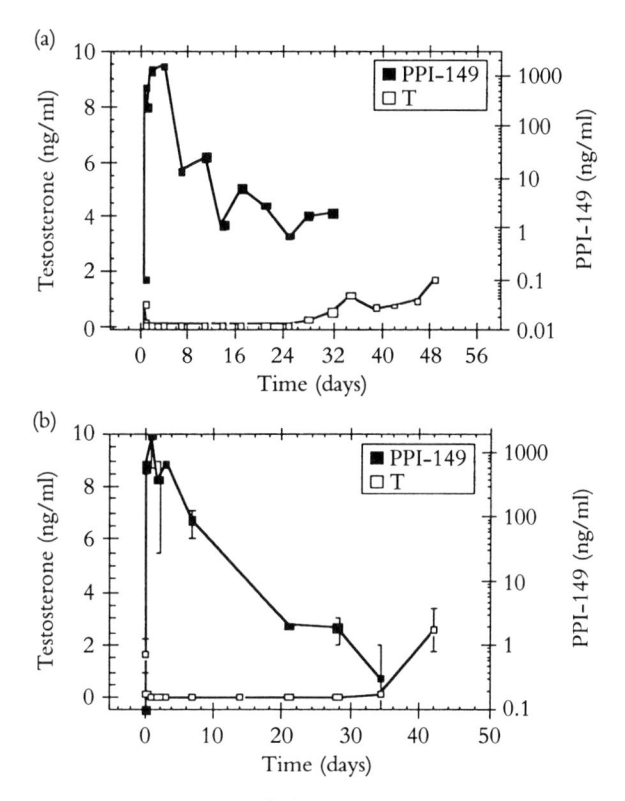

Figure 4 Long-term suppression of plasma testosterone (T) in the intact dog (a) and rat (b) by a single subcutaneous injection of abarelix depot (PPI-149) (3 mg/kg)

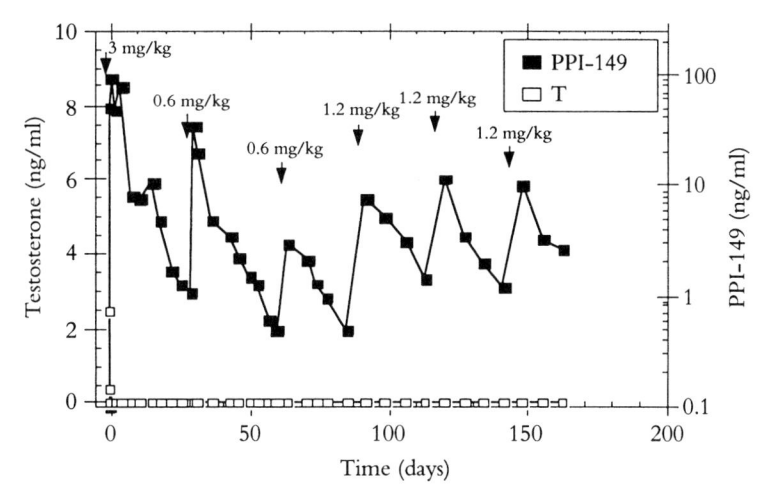

Figure 5 Long-term suppression of plasma testosterone (T) in the intact dog by multiple subcutaneous injections of abarelix depot (PPI-149) (1.2–3 mg/kg)

pharmacological effect of abarelix was reflected in reduced size and morphological regression of the testes, ovaries and accessory glands in males and females.

The authors pointed out that abarelix depot was the first long-acting formulation of a GnRH antagonist capable of providing sustained suppression of plasma testosterone levels, allowing monthly administration. This formulation has appropriate pharmacokinetics and pharmacodynamics for use in therapies requiring suppression of gonadal hormones in men and women. These results are now to be compared with those obtained in the rat with the recently disclosed FE200486.

PRESENTATION BY HUTCHISON AND COLLEAGUES [17]

Preclinical data on azaline B were reported by Shangold and co-workers in 1995[8]. The peptide was shown to be potent, long acting and safe in a number of animal species. These rigorous studies promised a very bright future for that peptide, as it compared favorably with other GnRH antagonists studied at the time.

The presentation by Hutchison was particularly enlightening, as it described several clinical investigations in a systematic fashion using azaline B in a 5% mannitol solution at different concentrations or as a controlled-release depot. The objectives were to demonstrate safety, tolerability and efficacy of subcutaneous administration in women and men. Since this group targeted endometriosis, one of their goals was to identify a regimen that regulated blood estradiol concentrations within a presumed therapeutic window, where serum estradiol levels would be low enough to ameliorate symptoms of endometriosis but high enough to prevent bone loss[9,10]. In men, the goal was to suppress testosterone to castrate range. Two types of formulation were evaluated, azaline B in solution in 5% mannitol and a controlled-release depot, and six clinical studies were presented, as outlined below.

A single ascending dose study in healthy postmenopausal women (0.75 mg/ml) showed a graded degree of inhibition of serum LH and a concomitant increase of duration of action with increasing doses of azaline B.

In healthy women with regular menstrual cycles, the dose of 60 μg/kg per week for 4 weeks was identified as being optimal for lowering the serum estradiol level to the presumed therapeutic range for treatment of endometriosis and uterine fibroids, as defined above (Figure 6). Unfortunately, it was determined that the concentration of the peptide used (0.75 mg/ml) required injection volumes (4–6 ml) that were unsuitable as a market formulation. At this dose and concentration of azaline

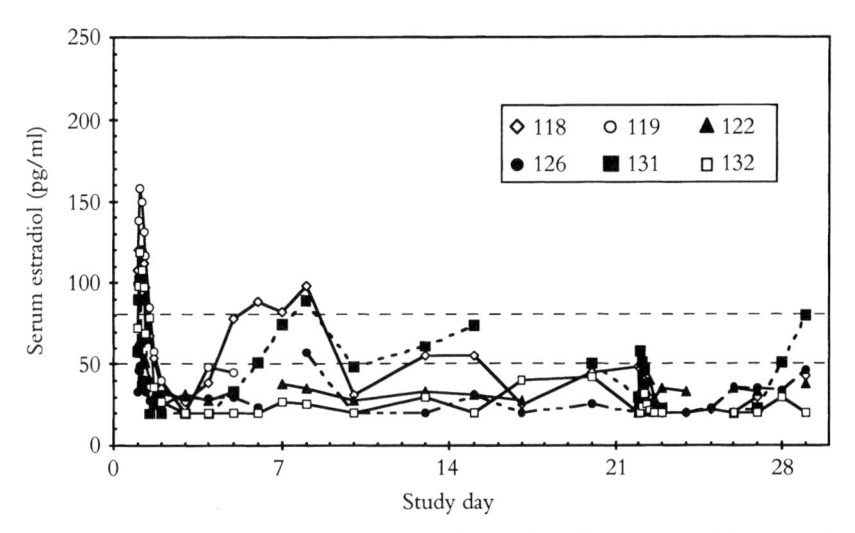

Figure 6 Serum concentration of estradiol in six healthy women (identified individually by number, 118, etc.) after subcutaneous administration of azaline B 60 µg/kg per week (0.75 mg/ml, 5% mannitol in water)

B, peak serum concentrations reached 10–15 ng/ml, which interrupted estradiol production, and subsided to 1–5 ng/ml, which maintained serum estradiol within or below the presumed therapeutic range.

A similar response was obtained when azaline B was administered subcutaneously at a dose of 640 µg/kg and a concentration of 5 mg/ml in healthy women. Suppression of estradiol to the therapeutic range was achieved for 1 month in six subjects out of seven, with higher doses of azaline B made possible by a higher concentration of injectate. Such a protocol still required three to five 2-ml injections and was judged to be practically unacceptable.

In healthy men, a single ascending dose study using 5 and 10 mg/ml of azaline B showed that, at the highest dose of 1280 µg/kg, serum testosterone was suppressed to < 50 ng/dl in only one of seven men. Because the serum pK of azaline B varied little (3–12 ng/ml), we concluded that there may be significant inter-subject variability in the set-point for suppression of testosterone to the castrate range. It became obvious that suppression of testosterone to the castrate range could not be achieved for a month using the 10 mg/ml formulation. This study led to the discovery that increasing the drug concentration from 5 to 10 mg/ml resulted, in fact, in reduced drug exposure. This is clearly shown in Figure 7; 320 µg/kg of azaline B at concentrations of 5 and 10 mg/ml yielded two distinct release levels, neither of which were high enough to achieve complete inhibition of testosterone secretion.

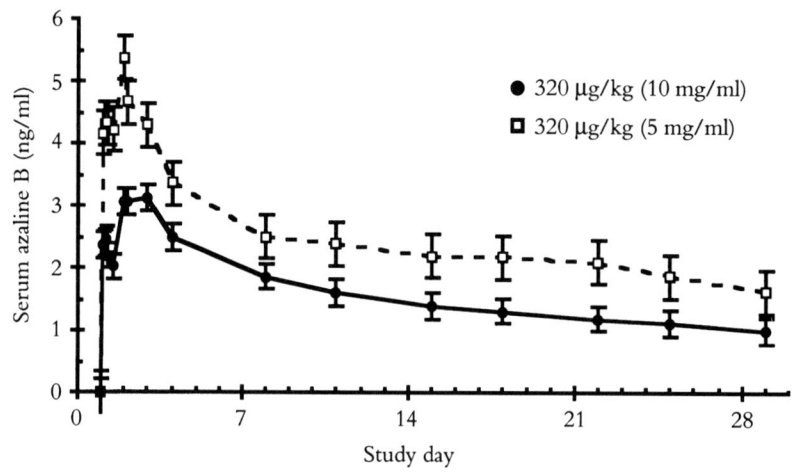

Figure 7 Serum concentration of azaline B after subcutaneous administration in men of azaline B 320 μg/kg at two concentrations (5 mg/ml and 10 mg/ml, 5% mannitol in water)

A likely explanation is that azaline B solutions form gels after subcutaneous administration and that the denser the gels (resulting from increased concentration) the less amenable they are to releasing the peptide. This bears witness to the limited solubility of azaline B.

The last two clinical studies in normal healthy women and men were carried out using a controlled-release formulation of azaline B in poly-DL- lactic/glycolic acid polymer (ProLease® azaline B) at a concentration of 15 mg/ml. The most promising results (inhibition of estradiol for 28 days in seven out of eight subjects) were obtained in women at a dose of 60 mg subcutaneously (two 2-ml injections per subject). In men, the same dose resulted in an insignificant lowering of serum testosterone.

The authors concluded that low solubility of azaline B, gelling and the inverse relationship between concentration and bioavailability prevented the use of 5% mannitol in water for azaline B concentrations greater than 10 mg/ml and that sufficient quantities of azaline B could not be administered in clinically acceptable volumes by the subcutaneous route. The same lack of solubility prevented loading ProLease (PLGA) polymer with more than 15 mg/ml of azaline B and therefore also required unacceptable injection volumes of this depot formulation.

Remarks

From a pragmatic point of view, it has always been accepted that delivery systems would have to be developed before peptide GnRH antagonists gained full acceptability. Abarelix depot and ganirelix depot are perfect examples of such an approach, whereby a readily available (read soluble) peptide is formulated in a slow-release preparation that will sustain delivery of the bioactive component at a rate sufficient to maintain bioactive levels in the circulation. Whether FE200486 has physicochemical properties such that it will not need to be formulated into a slow-release preparation for human therapies, as suggested by preclinical data, remains to be seen.

It is not clear at this point from the data presented whether any of these peptides and peptide preparations will inhibit gonadal functions reliably for periods of 1 month or more in humans after a single injection. Here, the two key words are 'reliably' and 'single'. Reliability indicates that all individuals will have their sex steroid levels maximally inhibited all the time. The issue of a single injection is also important because of the need for the peptide formulations described so far to be administered more often at the beginning of treatment corresponding to a 'loading period', of which I do not have a good understanding.

On the positive side, most of the analogues that were described were safe at the proposed dosages for therapeutic usage, although no long-term toxicology data were presented.

Interestingly, the question of cost of the drug was not addressed, suggesting that it is no longer an issue. Another positive aspect was the fact that the reliability of delivery systems was not addressed either. Does this mean that the technology in its infancy 6 years ago has been mastered for the handling of peptides? This could have a tremendous impact on other peptide drugs that, although very safe and very potent, may suffer from a lack of long duration of action.

On everyone's mind, however, was the question of when an orally active GnRH antagonist would become available. While it is obvious that oral administration of a drug is most convenient, I always like to make the point that compliance is much less of a problem with administration of a 1–3-month depot as compared to a daily or twice-daily pill. It was also not clear which indications would profit most from a daily administration of a GnRH antagonist, especially if, for some of the peptides described here, duration of action is proportional to dose and recovery observed upon disappearance of the drug in the bloodstream. One definite conclusion, however, is that good oral bioavailability (> 30%) is out of the question for decapeptides. This brings us to the forefront of current activities in the field of orally active GnRH antagonists.

PRESENTATION BY RIVIER AND COLLEAGUES [15]

Development of orally active peptides is still in its infancy; major roadblocks range from the instability of the bioactive component to enzymes, to problems associated with gut adsorption and elimination.

With the availability of the cloned GnRH receptor, a large number of companies have developed screening programs for small molecules that bind to this receptor. While there are several patents covering such molecules, only one promising mimetic has been described in the literature. With an affinity of 0.2 nmol/l on cloned human receptor-bearing cell lines, T98475 was described as having good oral bioavailability. The approach of my laboratory has been quite different and aimed first at identifying the bioactive conformation of GnRH antagonists. The hypothesis was that if we could identify constrained analogues with high potency, their nuclear magnetic resonance (NMR) structure would have to be that of the bioactive conformation. It is believed that a refined model of the bioactive conformation of GnRH antagonists can be used for the rational design of non-peptide, orally active molecules.

Little is known of the bioactive conformation of peptide hormones for a number of reasons; peptide hormones are notoriously flexible in solution, their receptors are particularly complex and there is strong evidence that receptor–ligand interaction leading to activation is a dynamic process. Receptor-competitive blockade, on the other hand, does not require ligand flexibility. In collaboration with R. J. Bienstock, J. Rizo, L. Gierasch and A. Hagler, we have described the NMR conformation of three constrained {cyclo(4-10), dicyclo(4-10/5-8) and dicyclo(4-10/5-5′-8)} GnRH antagonists, which all included a β-turn encompassing residues 5–8 and a less-defined turn around the residue at the 2 position[11–14]. The precise location of the N-terminal tripeptide with respect to the rest of the molecule remained unclear, owing to the rotational freedom between the two regions. The NMR conformations of the newly discovered dicyclo(1-1′-5/4-10) (Koerber, Hoeger and Rizo, submitted for publication) and dicyclo(1-8/4-10) GnRHs determined by Rizo and Gierasch now allow unequivocal positioning of the two parts of the molecule relative to each other. We have determined the commonly available conformations of these antagonists that are consistent with NMR data and have generated a consensus structure, which represents a single bioactive conformation (Figure 8). We have used it in the design of a tribetide library (tri-aminoglycine scaffold) that binds to the GnRH receptor with high affinity. Additionally, we have used this model to test its compatibility with the structure of the non-peptide T98475, which was recently described as having high affinity for the GnRH receptor. In the course of the latter

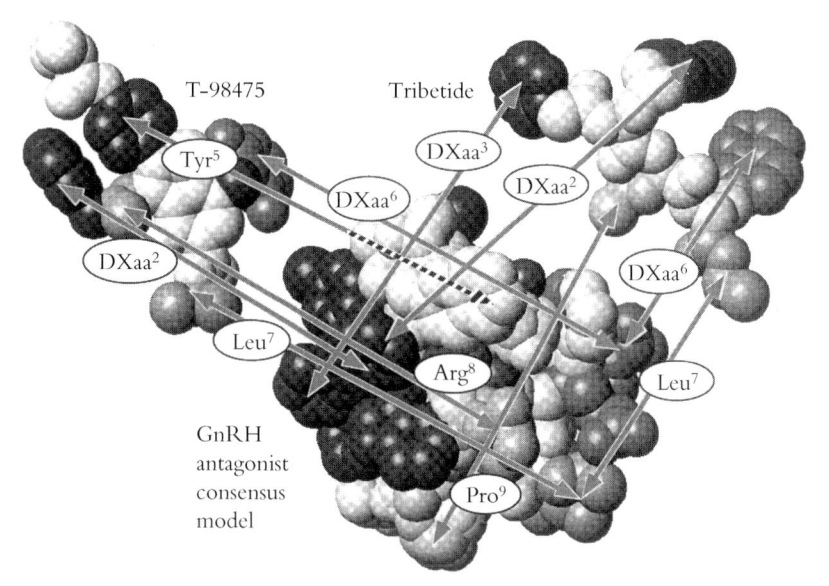

Figure 8 Structural correlations of space-filling models of T98475 and the Salk tribetide compound with the GnRH antagonist consensus model. The consensus model is represented by the four GnRH antagonists superimposed en masse to fit the individual NMR constraints and the group consensus forced constraint. The gray scale runs from dark gray to light gray in the order DXaa^2, DXaa^3, Tyr^5, DXaa^6, Leu^7, Arg^8, Pro^9; atoms not considered in the correlation are the lightest shade of gray

study, we identified two contact points not identified by the authors, suggesting that our model could have predictive value. Our model showed that T98475 interacts with the GnRH receptor at the same place where peptide GnRH antagonists act. This may not be a necessity for all peptide and non-peptide analogues. Beckers and colleagues [71] presented docking models for GnRH ligands based on site-specific mutants of the human GnRH receptor. Because the ligands seem to interact with residues embedded in the membrane, it will be some time before these hypotheses are verified by spectroscopic or X-ray data. In the meantime, I expect these models to inspire chemists in their design of small bioactive molecules and I am sure that the next few years will see a blossoming of the non-peptide GnRH field. Further developments will definitely take the uncharted path of non-peptide, combinatorially derived GnRH ligands. These new molecules will benefit tremendously during their development as drugs from the significant experience gained from the peptide predecessors.

In conclusion, attractive physicochemical properties of new antagonists have been identified and new proprietary formulations of water-soluble (> 50 mg/ml) and safe GnRH antagonists effective for about 1 month have been tested successfully in humans. The question therefore is not whether a peptide antagonist will gain drug status but rather for which indication(s) it will be used. The analogues or formulations that will ultimately prevail in the marketplace will probably be dictated by additional forces other than those described in this meeting. Also, non-peptide GnRH antagonists may rapidly enter the market. It is unlikely that these will be used for the same indications as the current long-acting depot preparations developed to address prostate cancer (and similar) indications. The new data presented at this meeting have therefore not necessarily raised the bar for GnRH non-peptide and orally active antagonists. I suspect that non-peptides will share different niches in an extremely wide field of possible indications. My prediction is, therefore, that a few peptidic long-acting preparations will be attractive for their safety, reliability, reversibility, specificity and, most importantly, their efficacy, which is superior to that of the GnRH agonists. Additionally, promising new formulations that allow protocols similar to those used for the agonists (single injections every 1–3 months) will be discovered that will not necessarily increase the overall cost of treatment.

ACKNOWLEDGEMENTS

My sincere thanks go to Drs Broqua, Hutchison, Molineaux and Boutignon and their colleagues who allowed me to present in this report some of their yet unpublished results. Work from my group was supported by NIH grant HD-13527 and the Hearst Foundation.

REFERENCES

1. Kutscher B, Bernd M, Beckers T, et al. Chemistry and molecular biology in the search for new LHRH antagonists. *Angew Chem Int Ed Engl* 1997; 36:2148–61
2. Rivier J, Porter J, Hoeger C, et al. Gonadotropin releasing hormone antagonists with N^ω-triazolyl-ornithine, -lysine or -para-aminophenylalanine residues at positions 5 and 6. *J Med Chem* 1992;35:4270–8
3. Molineaux CJ, Sluss PM, Bree MP, et al. Suppression of plasma gonadotropins by abarelix, a potent new LHRH antagonist. *Mol Urol* 1998;2:265–8
4. Nestor JJ Jr, Tahilramani R, Ho TL, et al. Design of luteinizing hormone releasing hormone antagonists with reduced potential for side effects. In Jung G, Bayer E, eds. *Peptides 1988*. Berlin: Walter de Gruyter, 1989:592–4
5. Bajusz S, Csernus VJ, Janaky T, et al. New antagonists of LHRH. II. Inhibition and potentiation of LHRH by closely related analogues. *Int J Pept Prot Res* 1988;32:425–35
6. Deghenghi R, Boutignon F, Wüthrich K, et al. Antarelix (EP 24332) a novel water soluble LHRH antagonist. *Biomed Pharmacother* 1993;47:107–10

7. Haviv F, Fitzpatrick TD, Nichols CJ, et al. The effect of NMeTyr[5] substitution in luteinizing hormone-releasing hormone antagonists. *J Med Chem* 1993; 36:928–33
8. Shangold GA, Campen CA, Hillips A, et al. Reproductive pharmacology and safety of azaline B: an overview of preclinical studies. In Filicori M, Flamigni C, eds. *Treatment with GnRH Analogs: Controversies and Perspectives; The Proceedings of a Satellite Symposium of the 15th World Congress on Fertility and Sterility*, Bologna, Italy. Carnforth, UK: Parthenon Publishing, 1996:93–100
9. Barbieri RL. Endometriosis and the estrogen threshold hypothesis. *J Reprod Med* 1998;34:287–92
10. Agarwal SK, Hamrang C, Henzl MR, et al. Nafarelin vs. leuprolide acetate depot for endometriosis. *J Reprod Med* 1997;42:413–23
11. Rizo J, Koerber SC, Bienstock RJ, et al. Conformational analysis of a highly potent, constrained gonadotropin-releasing hormone antagonist. I. Nuclear magnetic resonance. *J Am Chem Soc* 1992;114:2852–9
12. Rizo J, Koerber SC, Bienstock RJ, et al. Conformational analysis of a highly potent, constrained gonadotropin-releasing hormone antagonist. II. Molecular dynamics simulations. *J Am Chem Soc* 1992;114:2860–71
13. Rizo J, Sutton RB, Breslau J, et al. A novel conformation in a highly potent, constrained gonadotropin releasing hormone antagonist. *J Am Chem Soc* 1996;118:970–6
14. Bienstock RJ, Rizo J, Koerber SC, et al. Conformational analysis of a highly potent dicyclic gonadotropin-releasing hormone antagonist by nuclear magnetic resonance and molecular dynamics. *J Med Chem* 1993;36:3265–73

BIBLIOGRAPHY

Abstracts of relevant papers presented at the 5th International Symposium on GnRH Analogues in Cancer and Human Reproduction

15. Peptidomimetics of GnRH antagonists: present status. J. Rivier, C. Hoeger, S. Koerber, *et al.*, USA
16. Pharmacology and pharmacokinetics of abarelix-depot, a novel, long-acting formulation of the GnRH antagonist abarelix. C.J. Molineaux, R.M. McGarr, S.M. Oliveira, M.L. Gefter, M.B. Garnick, USA
17. Clinical pharmacology of azaline B. J. Hutchison, S. Liao, J. Smith, A. Phillips, USA
18. Pharmacological profile of FE200486, a potent, water soluble and long acting GnRH antagonist. P. Broqua, A. Aebi, G.C. Jiang, J. Stalewski, G. Semple, K. Akinsanya, R. Haigh, P. Rivière, J. Rivier, M.L. Aubert, J.L. Junien, Switzerland, USA and UK
71. Ligand binding and signal transduction by site-specific mutants of the human GnRH receptor. S.H. Hoffmann, H. Reiländer, R. Kühne, T. Reissmann, T. Beckers, Germany
78. Long-lasting suppression of plasma testosterone by Antarelix®-Depot: a sustained release preparation of the superantagonist teverelix. F. Boutignon, H. Touchet, F. Moine, D. Mallardé, S. David, R. Deghenghi, France

3
The use of GnRH antagonists in assisted reproduction technologies

R. E. Felberbaum and K. Diedrich

INTRODUCTION

We are living in exciting days at the moment. After having been used in extensive phase II and phase III trials, two gonadotropin releasing hormone (GnRH) antagonists of the newest generation, cetrorelix (Cetrotide®; ASTA Medica AG, Frankfurt/Main, Germany) and ganirelix (Orgalutran®; Organon, Oss, The Netherlands) are to be introduced to the market. Both seem to have solved the typical problems of former generations of GnRH antagonists, such as histamine release and anaphylactoid reactions, which had hampered further clinical development. Both GnRH antagonists of the newest generation have been incorporated successfully into protocols for controlled ovarian hyperstimulation (COH) for the avoidance of premature luteinization. Cetrorelix has been used in both a multiple-dose and a single-dose protocol, but ganirelix has been used only in the multiple-dose setting to date. Pregnancy rates obtained were comparable to those obtained in long agonistic protocols. It can therefore be assumed that the introduction of cetrorelix and ganirelix into the market will have an important impact on the attitude of clinicians towards COH for assisted reproduction. Without doubt we are standing at the verge of a new era in assisted reproduction technologies (ART)[1].

GnRH AGONISTS: STILL THE GOLD STANDARD FOR COH?

In some respects, the use of GnRH agonists for the purposes of COH marks the beginning of modern management within assisted reproduction. Premature luteinizing hormone (LH) surges had been responsible for a reduced effectiveness of ovarian stimulation by human menopausal gonadotropin (hMG) in an *in vitro* fertilization (IVF) program. At the same time, they negatively affected oocyte and embryo quality and thus the pregnancy rates obtained[2,3]. The introduction of agonist treatment has remedied most of these drawbacks, and the rate of stimulated cycles that must be terminated has been reduced to about 2%. Induction of ovulation has become possible to plan so that the psychological pressure on patients and physicians has been eased to some extent. Suppression of endogenous hormone production by GnRH analogues (GnRHa) followed by hMG stimulation has developed from second-line into first-line therapy. Different treatment schedules are currently applied, including the so-called 'long protocol', which aims at complete pituitary suppression, and the 'short' and 'ultrashort' protocols, in which the initial flare-up of gonadotropins is used for ovarian stimulation[4,5]. Among these protocols, the long protocol is generally the most effective and is most often used. In Germany, more than 70% of all stimulated cycles for ART are implemented according to the long protocol[6,7]. The long protocol has become the standard method in most major centers. In this setting, complete desensitization of the pituitary gland is aimed at before stimulation with human gonadotropins – urinary or recombinant – commences. The long agonistic protocol for COH has therefore become the gold standard, and any new attitude towards controlled ovarian stimulation has to be compared in its results with those obtained in the long agonistic protocol.

GnRH ANTAGONISTS

In parallel with the development of GnRH agonists, other analogues were synthesized which also bind to the pituitary GnRH receptors but are not functional in inducing the release of gonadotropins. These compounds are far more complex than GnRH agonists, with modifications in the molecular structure not only at positions 6 and 10, but also at positions 1, 2, 3 and 8. In comparison with the GnRH agonists, the pharmacological mechanism by which GnRH antagonists suppress the liberation of gonadotropins is completely different. The agonists act on chronic administration through down-regulation of receptors and desensitization of the gonadotropic cells, whereas the antagonists bind competitively to the receptors and thereby prevent the endogenous GnRH from exerting its stimulatory effects on the pituitary cells, avoiding any 'flare-up' effect. Within hours the secretion of gonadotropins is reduced[8]. This mechanism of action is dependent on the equilibrium between endogenous GnRH and the applied antagonist. The effect of the antagonists is highly dose dependent, in contrast to that of the agonists[9]. GnRH antagonists fail to block gonadotropin secretion when administered together with pulsatile GnRH at a dose that is sufficiently high to override receptor blockade[10]. This made it possible to restore ovulatory cycles in monkeys during antagonist treatment by the pulsatile administration of native GnRH[11].

In the first generation of GnRH antagonists, allergic side-effects due to an induced histamine release hampered the clinical development of these compounds[12,13]. Modern GnRH antagonists such as ganirelix or cetrorelix seem to have solved these problems.

Ganirelix and cetrorelix: characteristics

Ganirelix is a third-generation GnRH antagonist with six substituted amino acids at positions 1, 2, 3, 6, 8 and 10 and a molecular weight of 1570. Ganirelix is presented as a sterile, ready-for-use solution for injection intended for subcutaneous administration. It induces a rapid, profound, reversible suppression of endogenous gonadotropins by competitive binding to the GnRH receptors in the pituitary gland. Ganirelix has a high aqueous solubility, a high absolute bioavailability (> 90%) and a relatively short elimination half-life of approximately 13 h. Accordingly, ganirelix is fully effective within 4 h and treatment discontinuation leads to an immediate recovery of the pituitary–gonadal axis. Ganirelix is well tolerated. Evaluation of safety data of approximately 800 patients treated with ganirelix revealed that none of the patients had to discontinue treatment because of a hypersensitivity reaction or because of a drug-related adverse experience [24].

Cetrorelix shows substituted amino acids at positions 1, 2, 3, 6 and 10. It also induces a rapid, profound and reversible suppression of gonadotropin secretion of the pituitary gland by competitive classic receptor blockade at the gonadotropic cells. Cetrorelix is fully effective within 8 h and its elimination half-life is about 36 h. A 3-mg dose of cetrorelix as an intermediate depot preparation is able to suppress endogenous LH secretion for about 96 h. Cetrorelix is well tolerated. A total of 2000 patients and healthy subjects have finished treatment with cetrorelix for different benign and malignant gynecological or urological indications. Single or multiple doses of 0.1 mg/day up to 10 mg/day for 9 months or for several years have been administered.

GnRH antagonists within COH

In 1991 Dittkoff and colleagues[14] showed that a GnRH antagonist applied for a short period was capable of suppressing the ovulation-inducing midcycle LH peak. They administered 50 μg of Nal-Glu per kilogram body weight per day for 4 days in the midcycle phase. The LH peak failed to occur, estradiol production came to a halt and follicular growth was interrupted. After the antagonists were discontinued, gonadal function normalized within days. Apparently, the antagonists neither depleted the follicle stimulating hormone (FSH) and LH stores of gonadotropic cells nor inhibited gonadotropin synthesis. Therefore, timely administration of GnRH antagonists in the late follicular phase of the cycle seemed to offer an interesting alternative in ovarian stimulation for IVF[15].

Extrapolating these results into a protocol of COH with hMG to avoid the onset of premature luteinization, the premature LH surge seems to be abolished both by daily administration of the modern GnRH antagonists cetrorelix or ganirelix from day 7 onward until ovulation induction, and by single administration at day 8[16,17]. The latter protocol has been applied only to cetrorelix so far, while ganirelix has been used only in the multiple-dose setting.

The importance of pilot studies

The successful use of sophisticated compounds such as cetrorelix or ganirelix in COH for ART was possible only because of important preclinical research and clinical pilot studies using second-generation antagonists such as Nal-Glu or antide. It was demonstrated that it was possible to inhibit the premature LH surge during COH by daily midcycle administration as well as by single-dose administration[14,15,18]. In fact, the first prospective randomized trial using a GnRH antagonist compared to an agonist in COH was performed by using Nal-Glu. This pilot trial suggested the superiority of GnRH antagonists for this purpose[19].

Dose-finding studies: ganirelix and cetrorelix

Cetrorelix: multiple-dose protocol

Starting on cycle day 2, patients have been treated in the multiple-dose protocol with 150 IU FSH and 150 IU LH per day. From cycle day 7 until ovulation induction, patients were treated in the early stages of developing this protocol with the rather high dosage of 3 mg cetrorelix per day, administered subcutaneously. On day 5 the dose of hMG was adjusted to the individual ovarian response of the patient to the stimulation, as assessed by estradiol values and measurement of follicles. This treatment was continued until induction of ovulation with 10 000 IU intramuscular human chorionic gonadotropin (hCG), given when the leading follicle reached a diameter of 18–20 mm, measured by transvaginal ultrasound, and when estradiol values indicated a satisfactory follicular response.

To elucidate the question of the dosage necessary for sufficient suppression of the pituitary gland at this critical moment of controlled ovarian hyperstimulation in two subsequent open phase II studies, three dosages were administered in accordance with the 'Lübeck protocol' and comparisons were made between the hormone profiles obtained, the number of oocytes retrieved, the fertilization rates and the consumption of hMG.

A total of 35 patients, all suffering from tubal infertility and no other infertility factors observed, were treated as described. No premature LH surge was observed (Figure 1). All cycles were evaluated. The mean courses in the three dosage groups of FSH and LH were quite similar with a profound suppression of LH and a less pronounced suppression of FSH, the latter observation probably due to the longer half-life in plasma of the injected FSH.

The fertilization rates of the recovered oocytes after conventional IVF were 45.3% in the 3-mg group, 53.2% in the 1-mg group and 67.7% in the 0.5-mg group, showing a clear tendency towards better results in the lower dosages. In the 3-mg group 106 oocytes were recovered and 30 embryos were obtained, 36.7% of them being excellent according to morphological microscopic criteria. In the 1-mg group 94 oocytes were collected and 28 embryos obtained, 53.6% being excellent. In the 0.5-mg group, 127 oocytes were recovered and 27 embryos were obtained, 37% of them being excellent (Table 1).

The average use of hMG ampules was 30 in the 3-mg group, 27 in the 1-mg group and 26 in the 0.5-mg group. These differences were not significant, but have to be compared with the higher number of ampules used in an agonistic long protocol[20].

Subsequent dose-finding studies using 0.5 mg cetrorelix per day, 0.25 mg cetrorelix per day and 0.1 mg cetrorelix per day proved the efficacy and safety of

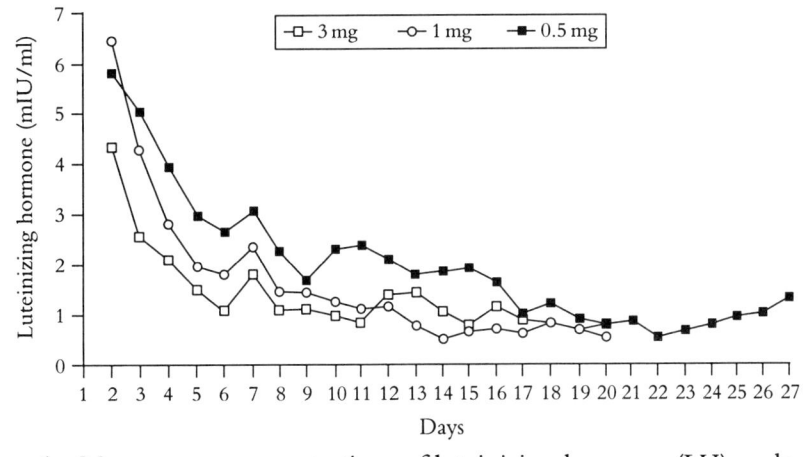

Figure 1 Mean serum concentrations of luteinizing hormone (LH) under controlled ovarian hyperstimulation with human menopausal gonadotropin and concomitant cetrorelix administration at various dosages (3 mg/day, 1 mg/day, 0.5 mg/day)

0.25 mg cetrorelix per day in avoiding premature LH surges, whereas, under 0.1 mg cetrorelix per day, premature LH surges were observed[21,22]. In these studies intracytoplasmic sperm injection (ICSI) for treatment of male subfertility of the husband was allowed, leading to fertilization rates within the range to be expected after normal oocyte maturation. There were no significant differences regarding two-pronuclei fertilization rates, increase in estradiol values, cleavage rate, clinical pregnancy rate per embryo transfer and implantation rate between the group treated with 0.5 mg cetrorelix per day and those patients treated with only 0.25 mg per day (Table 2). The clinical pregnancy rates per transfer were 30.7% in the 0.5-mg group

Table 1 Recovered oocytes, fertilization rate, number and quality of embryos after controlled ovarian hyperstimulation with human menopausal gonadotropin and concomitant cetrorelix treatment at three different dosages (3 mg/day, 1 mg/day, 0.5 mg/day) for *in vitro* fertilization

	3 mg	*1 mg*	*0.5 mg*
Number of oocytes	106	94	127
Fertilization rate (%)	45.3	53.2	67.7
Number of embryos	30	28	27
Excellent embryos (%)	36.7	53.6	37

Table 2 Stimulation and outcome of intracytoplasmic sperm injection in patients treated with human menopausal gonadotropin (hMG) and concomitant midcycle cetrorelix at 0.5 and 0.25 mg/day

	0.5 mg/day	*0.25 mg/day*
Number of patients	32	30
Number of hMG ampules	35	33
Duration of hMG treatment (days)	11	10
Number of follicles > 15 mm on the day of hCG administration	10	10
Estradiol on the day of hCG administration (pg/ml)	2122	2491
Fertilization rate (%)	55	59
Cleavage rate (%)	78	76
Clinical pregnancy rate (%)	31	30

hCG, human chorionic gonadotropin

and 29.6% in the 0.25-mg group. Interestingly, about 16% of the patients treated in this study with 0.5 mg cetrorelix per day and 10% of those treated with only 0.25 mg per day showed a significant rise in LH concentrations during the follicular phase, while progesterone concentrations remained low. These patients showed a significantly lower cleavage rate, and no pregnancy occurred in this subgroup of patients. As these patients showed higher estradiol concentrations than patients who did not have a rise of LH, these findings may suggest that an earlier administration of the antagonist may be necessary in high responders to avoid the LH rise, which may compromise the quality and maturity of the recovered oocytes[22].

Cetrorelix: single-dose protocol

In parallel with the multiple-dose administration, a different protocol for administration of GnRH antagonists within COH was developed by the French investigators Olivennes and colleagues[16,23] in which the compound is used in a dosage of 2 mg or 3 mg as single or dual administration around day 9. In this protocol, the antagonist is injected at the time that the estradiol concentration reaches 150–200 pg/ml and the follicle size is > 14 mm, which is usually the case on day 8 or 9 of the cycle. These investigators did not observe premature LH rises in any of the cycles studied and published. The injection of 3 mg cetrorelix on the *jour fixe* of the 8th day of the cycle was capable of preventing LH surges in the patients treated by suppressing LH secretion for about 96 h, introducing a very simple treatment protocol. Clinical pregnancy rates of over 30% per transfer were reported, which sound very promising.

Ganirelix: multiple-dose protocol

Ganirelix was tested within the frame of a clinical phase II study in combination with recombinant FSH. In contrast to urinary compounds, these preparations are free of LH activity. Their effectiveness within COH according to the long protocol has been proved. Even after down-regulation of the pituitary gland, endogenous LH secretion seems to be sufficient for normal ovarian sexual steroid biosynthesis. However, extreme suppression of LH secretion by high doses of GnRH antagonists could cause problems according to the two cell/two gonadotropin hypothesis of follicular estrogen production[24]. Causing a situation very similar to that in patients classified as infertile according to the World Health Organization (WHO) grade I, ovarian stimulation with pure FSH depleted of any LH activity could induce follicular growth in the absence of any estrogen secretion, as was described in these patients[25]. It is the merit of this prospective, multicenter, double-blind, dose-finding, phase II study with ganirelix to have elucidated this question and demonstrating the correctness of the two cell/two gonadotropin theory. In this study, ganirelix was administered according to the multiple-dose protocol ('Lübeck protocol') at six different dosages (0.0625 mg/day, 0.125 mg/day, 0.25 mg/day, 0.5 mg/day, 1 mg/day and 2 mg/day). While in the lower dosages estradiol secretion was normal and sufficient, injecting 2 mg ganirelix subcutaneously per day showed almost no increase of the estradiol secretion. In some cases even the follicles did not grow, an observation that still awaits its scientific explanation. The treatment outcome in the 0.25-mg group was an overwhelming success, showing a clinical pregnancy rate of 40.3% per transfer. With an increase in the dosage of ganirelix, the pregnancy rates dropped and the abortion rates rose. Therefore, 0.25 mg was defined as the minimal effective dose to be administered according to the multiple-dose protocol[26].

Results of phase III studies

Ganirelix

The GnRH antagonist ganirelix was applied in a multicenter, open-label, randomized study to assess its safety and efficacy in women undergoing COH with recombinant FSH according to the multiple-dose protocol described above. The study had been designed as a non-inferiority study using a long protocol of buserelin (intranasal) and recombinant FSH as a reference treatment. In total, 730 subjects were randomized in a treatment ratio of 2 : 1 (ganirelix : buserelin). Evaluation of all safety data indicated that the ganirelix regimen was safe and well tolerated. The overall incidence of ovarian hyperstimulation syndrome was only 2.4% in the ganirelix group and 5.9% in the reference group. The median duration of GnRHa treatment was 5 days in the ganirelix group and 26 days in the buserelin group, whereas the median total FSH dose was 1500 IU and 1800 IU, respectively. In addition, in the ganirelix group the duration of stimulation was 1 day shorter. During the treatment with ganirelix, the incidence of LH rises, as defined in this study (LH ≥ 10 IU/l) was 2.8% versus 1.3% during FSH stimulation in the buserelin group. At the day on which ovulation was triggered by hCG, the mean number of follicles of > 11 mm was 10.7 and 11.8 and the median serum estradiol levels were 1190 pg/ml and 1700 pg/ml for the ganirelix and buserelin groups, respectively. The mean numbers of oocytes per pick-up were respectively 9.1 and 10.4. The fertilization rates were equal in both groups (62.1%) and the same mean numbers of embryos (2.2) were replaced. The mean implantation rates as reported were 15.7% in the ganirelix group and 21.8% in the buserelin group. The clinical pregnancy rates per transfer were 25.1% and 31.7% in the ganirelix and buserelin groups, respectively [26] (Table 3).

Table 3 Controlled ovarian hyperstimulation for assisted reproduction with recombinant follicle stimulating hormone and concomitant midcycle ganirelix administration at 0.25 mg/day. Results of a multicenter prospective randomized phase III study

	Ganirelix	Buserelin
Number of patients	463	237
Number of patients who reached the day of hCG administration	448	224
Number of patients with oocyte pick-up	440	221
Number of patients with embryo transfer	399	208
Cancellation rate (%)	13.8	12.6
LH rises during treatment (%)	2.8	1.3
Days of analogue treatment	5	26
Fertilization rate (%)	62.1	62.1
Clinical pregnancy rate per embryo transfer (%)	25.1	31.7
Overall incidence of OHSS (%)	2.4	5.9

hCG, human chorionic gonadotropin; LH, luteinizing hormone; OHSS, ovarian hyperstimulation syndrome

Cetrorelix

Multiple-dose protocol In a multicenter prospective randomized phase III study, 188 patients were treated with cetrorelix with its minimal effective dosage of 0.25 mg/day according to the multiple-dose protocol. These were compared with 85 patients treated according to the long protocol, using buserelin (600 µg/day) as a nasal spray for desensitization of the pituitary gland. While 181 patients reached the day of hCG injection in the cetrorelix group (96.3%), this was only the case in 77 of the buserelin group (90.6%), reflecting a lower cancellation rate in the antagonist group. The duration of analogue treatment was only 5.7 days in the cetrorelix group, but 26.6 days in the buserelin group. The numbers of follicles of > 20 mm on the day of hCG injection were 1.9 and 1.8, the numbers of small follicles of 11–14 mm were 3.2 and 4.3 in the cetrorelix group and the buserelin group, respectively. The difference in small follicles reached statistical significance ($p = 0.01$). The serum concentration of 17β-estradiol on the day of hCG administration was 1625 pg/ml in patients treated with cetrorelix and 2082 pg/ml in those treated with buserelin, showing a statistically significant difference ($p < 0.01$). The difference in number of ampules used per cycle, although being small (23.6 ampules in the cetrorelix group vs. 25.6 ampules in the busrelin group), was statistically significant

($p < 0.01$). The fertilization rates were very similar (53.6% in the cetrorelix group vs. 52.9 in the buserelin group), while the cleavage rate was clearly higher in the antagonist group than in the group treated with buserelin according to the long agonistic protocol (89.5% vs. 79.9%). The clinical pregnancy rate (intrauterine pregnancies with documented heart activity of the embryo) in the antagonist group was 26.1% per transfer and in the buserelin group was 32.8%. However, this difference was not statistically significant. The incidence of severe ovarian hyperstimulation syndrome (OHSS) WHO grade II–III was significantly higher in the buserelin group (five out of 77 patients; 6.5%) than in the cetrorelix group (two out of 181 patients; 1.1%) ($p = 0.026$ according to Fisher's exact test) [28] (Table 4).

In a prospective non-randomized study a total of 346 women with normal ovulatory functions were stimulated according to the multiple-dose protocol with

Table 4 Controlled ovarian hyperstimulation for assisted reproduction with human menopausal gonadotropin (hMG) and concomitant midcycle cetrorelix administration at 0.25 mg/day. Results of a multicenter prospective randomized phase III study

	Cetrorelix	*Buserelin*
Number of patients	188	85
Days of analogue treatment	57	266
Number of patients who reached the day of hCG administration	181 (96.3%)	77 (90.6%)
hMG ampules (*n*)	23.6	25.6
Estradiol (pg/ml) on the day of hCG administration	1625 ± 836	2082 ± 1049
Number of patients with oocyte pick-up	178	77
COC (*n*)	1398	816
Fertilization rate (%)	53.6	52.9
Cleavage rate (%)	89.5	79.9
Number of embryo transfers	157	67
Clinical pregnancy rate per embryo transfer (%)	26.1	32.8
Number of ectopic pregnancies	1	0
Number of deliveries per embryo transfer	30 (19.1%)	17 (25.3%)
Number of embryos replaced	343	147
Number of children born per embryo replaced	37 (10.8 %)	19 (12.9%)
Incidence of OHSS grades II–III (%)	1.1	6.5

hCG, human chorionic gonadotropin; COC, cumulus–oocyte complexes; OHSS, ovarian hyperstimulation syndrome (hMG) for COH, also using 0.25 mg cetrorelix per day. A total of 333 patients (96.2%) reached the day of hCG administration, and 324 (93.6%) underwent oocyte pick-up. A mean of 25.2 ampules of hMG was applied for a mean of 10.4 days. Cetrorelix was administered for a mean time lapse of 5.7 days. A total of 160 patients were submitted to the IVF procedure and 173 to ICSI. A mean of 8.5 cumulus–oocyte complexes per patient was obtained in the IVF group and 9.3 in the ICSI group. Only from two patients undergoing oocyte pick-up could no cumulus–oocyte complexes be obtained. The mean normal fertilization rate was 60% in the IVF group and 59% in the ICSI group. By replacing a mean of 2.7 embryos in 297 embryo transfers, 72 pregnancies were achieved, reflecting an ongoing clinical pregnancy rate of 24% per transfer. Only three LH rises (≥ 10 mIU/ml) with increase of progesterone secretion (≥ 1 ng/ml) were observed after initiation of cetrorelix administration, producing an incidence of premature luteinization of 0.9%. The abortion rate was 15%. The incidence of serious ovarian hyperstimulation syndrome (grade III) was as low as 0.6% [28] (Table 5).

Single-dose protocol   A total of 115 patients have been treated according to the single-dose protocol in a prospective, randomized phase III study, using 3 mg of cetrorelix injected on day 8 of the cycle. Their results were compared with those of 39 patients treated with triptorelin as a depot preparation according to the long protocol. No LH surge occurred after the cetrorelix administration in any of the patients studied. A higher number of oocytes (12.8 vs. 9.2) and embryos (7.5 vs. 5.4) were obtained in the patients from the triptorelin group. The percentages of mature oocytes (78.5% in the cetrorelix group vs. 81.7% in the triptorelin group) and the fertilization rate (50.5% in the cetrorelix group vs. 54.7% in the triptorelin group) were not statistically different. As in the case of the multiple-dose protocol, the pregnancy rate was slightly more favorable in the agonist group (28.2% per attempt; 27.3% per embryo transfer) than in the cetrorelix group (22.6% per attempt; 21.2% per embryo transfer). However, these differences were again not statistically significant. The incidence of OHSS (WHO grade II–III) was remarkably lower in those patients who had been treated with cetrorelix (1.8%) than in those who had been stimulated according to the long protocol using triptorelin depot (5.6%). While in the cetrorelix group only a mean of 24.3 ampules hMG was used, the mean amount of gonadotropins necessary for successful stimulation was 35.6 ampules per cycle. Interstingly, in all of the patients who had started to show a rise in LH on day 8, when cetrorelix was to be administered, the LH rise could be reduced by the administration of the antagonist. None of these cycles had to be cancelled and pregnancies also occurred [27] (Table 6).

Table 5 Cumulus–oocyte complexes (COCs), fertilization rates, embryos, quality of embryos, implantation rates, pregnancy rates and abortion rates following controlled ovarian hyperstimulation for *in vitro* fertilization (IVF) and intracytoplasmic sperm injection (ICSI) with human menopausal gonadotropin and concomitant midcycle cetrorelix administration at 0.25 mg/day. Results of a multicenter prospective non-randomized phase III study

	IVF	ICSI*	Total
Patients (*n*)	149	173	322
COC	1279	1692	2971
Mature oocytes			
n	811		
% of COC[†]	63.0 ± 35.6		
Metaphase II oocytes			
n		1252	
% of COC[†]		74.7 ± 25.0%	
Fertilization rate (%)[††]	60.4 ± 26.3	58.2 ± 24.5	59.2 ± 25.3
Total embryos	605	647	1252
Excellent embryos			
n	211	219	430
% of all	34.9	33.8	34.3
Good embryos			
n	281	298	579
% of all	46.4	46.1	46.2
Fair embryos			
n	113	130	243
% of all	18.7	20.1	19.4
Patients with embryo transfer	134	163	297
Clinical pregnancies	30	40	70
Pregnancy rate per embryo transfer (%)	22.4	24.5	23.6
Babies born after embryo transfer	33	45	78
Babies born/replaced embryos (%)	9.3	10.2	9.8
Miscarriages			
n	6	6	12
%	20.0	15.0	17.1

*In 11 patients IVF and ICSI were performed; [†]patient-based ratios; [‡]patients included only if total number of obtained oocytes > 0

Table 6 Controlled ovarian hyperstimulation for assisted reproduction with human menopausal gonadotropin (hMG) and single-dose injection of 3 mg cetrorelix on cycle day 8 compared with treatment with triptorelin as a depot preparation. Results of a multicenter prospective randomized phase III study

	Cetrorelix	Triptorelin depot
Number of patients	115	39
hCG administered (%)	98.3	92.3
Patients with OPU (%)	98.3	92.3
Patients with embryo transfer (%)	86.1	84.6
Incidence of LH surges	2.6	2.6
Days of stimulation	9.4	10.7
Number of hMG ampules	24.3	35.6
Estradiol (pg/ml) on the day of hCG administration	1786 ± 808	2549 ± 1194
COC per patient	9.2	10.7
Fertilization rate (%)	50.5	54.7
Clinical pregnancy rate per embryo transfer (%)	21.2	27.3
Babies born per embryos replaced (%)	10.6	13.3
OHSS grades II–III (%)	1.8	5.6

hCG, human chorionic gonadotropin; OPU, oocyte pick-up; LH, luteinizing hormone; COC, cumulus–oocyte complexes; OHSS, ovarian hyperstimulation syndrome

GnRH antagonist levels in plasma and follicular fluid

For both GnRH antagonists, ganirelix as well as cetrorelix, it was shown that the plasma and follicular fluid levels in COH according to the multiple-dose protocol using the minimal effective dosage of 0.25 mg/day were in most cases below the levels of quantification. At the time of embryo transfer, no GnRH antagonist could be measured in plasma samples. Since in reproductive medicine medication levels as low as possible should be obtained, this observation seems to be another advantage of GnRH antagonists in COH compared to GnRH agonists, e.g. depot preparations [24, 30, 100].

Direct effects of GnRH antagonists used for COH

Administered in a multiple-dose fashion in the midcycle phase, the minimal effective daily dose of cetrorelix (0.25 mg/day) does not impair either estradiol secretion *in vivo* or follicular development using hMG or recombinant FSH for COH. However, the importance of GnRH receptors on the granulosa–lutein cells and possible direct extrapituitary actions of the GnRH antagonists are still a matter of debate, although the function of these receptors remains unknown. It was shown in the rat that GnRH antagonists are able to inhibit gonadal steroid secretion *in vitro*[27,28]. Therefore, a negative impact of GnRH antagonists on the gonadal steroid secretion during COH or in the luteal phase in IVF cycles cannot be ruled out. However, all studies presented to date have demonstrated that in human granulosa–lutein cells neither agonists nor antagonists have any effect on sex steroid secretion in the presence or absence of hCG [101]. It was concluded that GnRH antagonists do not extert any significant actions on ovarian steroidogenesis *in vitro* and therefore their introduction into protocols of COH is unlikely to induce adverse effects on ovarian function.

Preserved pituitary response under GnRH antagonist treatment

On the basis of the mechanism of competitive binding, it is possible to modulate the degree of hormone suppression by the dose of antagonist to be administered. This preservation of the pituitary response due to competitive mechanisms was clearly demonstrated by using a GnRH test during GnRH antagonist treatment. At 3 h before injecting hCG for ovulation induction, 25 µg of GnRH was administered in patients treated with 1 mg cetrorelix per day or 3 mg cetrorelix per day. Blood samples for LH measurement were taken before and 30 min after GnRH treatment. The mean increase was 10 mIU/ml for the 3-mg group, while the average maximum concentration of serum LH in the 1-mg group was about 32.5 mIU/ml. These results were highly significant[9]. They could open new paths in the treatment of patients at higher risk for developing OHSS, as it would allow the avoidance in some cases of deleterious effects of hCG administration. Ovulation induction is possible by GnRH agonists or native GnRH itself under antagonistic treatment. This could help to lower the incidence rate of early-onset OHSS [29].

Ongoing discussions

The fact that, in all prospective comparative multicenter studies, there were slightly more favorable pregnancy rates observed in the control groups treated with agonists according to the long protocol than in the patient groups treated with GnRH antagonists caused concern and open discussions. Although no statistically significant differences were obtained, and although single-center or bicenter trials had shown equivalent or even better results in the antagonist groups, there may be possible negative effects on the implantation process [37]. However, as the percentage of good and excellent embryos obtained after COH using GnRH antagonists is quite high, possible effects on the condition of the endometrium should be properly observed. There is an important demand for *in vitro* studies regarding the implantation process using GnRH both agonists and antagonists. It seems essential to emphasize that, even in properly driven phase III studies, an important bias regarding study population characteristics, treatment indications and incidences of primary or secondary infertility may jeopardize the results obtained. This was demonstrated very clearly in the multiple-dose phase III study using cetrorelix [28]. In this study, only two centers showed significantly higher pregnancy rates in the buserelin group, but also significant differences in patient characteristics, while all other centers involved in the study obtained equivalent or even better results in the antagonist group.

New concepts in COH related to the use of GnRH antagonists

For almost a decade the association of GnRH agonists and hMG/recombinant FSH has been the routine procedure. This regimen includes mostly a profound downregulation, long duration of treatment, a substantial consumption of hMG ampules and a luteal phase deficiency. The use of GnRH antagonists opens new treatment modalities. The natural cycle and the association of clomiphene citrate/hMG are possible options to be used[29]. Although these treatment modalities still have to be called experimental, a review of the preliminary data indicates a pregnancy rate of 30% (with clomiphene citrate/hMG antagonist). The use of GnRH antagonists allows new strategies to be used which have to be tested extensively [31].

CONCLUSIONS

Modern GnRH antagonists such as cetrorelix and ganirelix have been proven to prevent premature LH surges reliably in controlled ovarian hyperstimulation for assisted reproductive technologies. Cetrorelix and ganirelix are safe and effective compounds. Owing to their distinct pharmacological mode of action, it was possible to achieve a significant reduction of treatment time as well as a reduction of the amount of gonadotropins necessary for successful stimulation. The fertilization rates and pregnancy rates are comparable to those obtained in agonistic protocols for ovarian stimulation. No allergic or hyperergic reactions occurred. Patient compliance was excellent. As all studies performed so far excluded patients with complex or difficult conditions such as polycystic ovarian disease, or low responders, experience and results have to be awaited in these special cases. In general, both the multiple-dose and the single-dose administration protocols seem to be appropriate. Whether GnRH antagonists will replace GnRH agonists in this indication remains an open question. Time will tell.

REFERENCES

1. Felberbaum RE, Ludwig M, Diedrich K. Are we on the verge of a new era in ART? *Hum Reprod* 1998;13:1778–80
2. Loumaye E. The control of endogenous secretion of LH by gonadotropin-releasing hormone agonists during ovarian hyperstimulation for *in vitro* fertilization and embryo transfer. *Hum Reprod* 1990;5:357–76
3. Stanger JD, Yovich JL. Reduced *in vitro* fertilization of human oocytes from patients with raised basal luteinizing hormone levels during the follicular phase. *Br J Obstet Gynaecol* 1985;92:385–93
4. Macnamee MC, Howles CM, Edwards RG, Taylor PJ, Elder KT. Short term luteinizing hormone-releasing hormone agonist treatment: prospective trial of a novel ovarian stimulation regimen for *in vitro* fertilization. *Fertil Steril* 1989;52:264–9
5. Loumaye E, de Cooman S, Anoma M, *et al*. Short term utilization of a gonadotropin releasing hormone agonist (buserelin) for induction of ovulation in an *in-vitro* fertilization program. *Ann NY Acad Sci* 1988;541:96–102
6. *Deutsches IVF-Register – Jahrbuch* 1996. Bundesgeschäftsstelle Bad Segeberg, Bismarckallee 116, 22353 Bad Segeberg
7. French IVF Registry. FIVNAT 1995 report. *Contracept Fertil Sex* 1995;24/9:694–9
8. Sommer L, Klingmüller D, Diedrich K. Effects of the GnRH antagonist cetrorelix in normal women. *Gynecol Endocrinol* 1993;7:2
9. Felberbaum RE, Reissmann T, Küpker W, *et al*. Preserved pituitary response under ovarian stimulation with hMG and GnRH-antagonists (cetrorelix) in women with tubal infertility. *Eur J Obstet Gynecol Reprod Biol* 1995;61:151–5
10. Dubourdieu S, Charbonnel B, d'Acremont MF. Effect of administration of a GnRH antagonist (Nal-Glu) during the preovulatory period: the luteinizing hormone surge requires the secretion of GnRH. *J Clin Endocrinol Metab* 1994;78:343–7
11. Gordon K, Danforth DR, Williams RF, Hodgen GD. A novel regimen of gonadotrophin-releasing hormone (GnRH) antagonist plus pulsatile GnRH: controlled restoration of gonadotrophin secretion and ovulation induction. *Fertil Steril* 1990;54:1140–5
12. Hahn DW, McGuire JL, Vale WW, Rivier J. Reproductive/endocrine and anaphylactoid properties of an LHRH antagonist (ORF-18260). *Life Sci* 1985;37:505–14
13. Reissmann T, Felberbaum R, Diedrich K, *et al*. Development and applications of luteinizing hormone-releasing hormone antagonists in the treatment of infertility: an overview. *Hum Reprod* 1995;10:1974–81
14. Dittkoff EC, Cassidenti DL, Paulson RJ, *et al*. The gonadotrophin-releasing hormone antagonist (Nal-Glu) acutely blocks the luteinizing hormone surge but allows for resumption of folliculogenesis in normal women. *Am J Obstet Gynecol* 1991;165:1811–17
15. Frydman R, Cornel C, de Ziegler D, *et al*. Prevention of premature luteinizing hormone and progesterone rise with a GnRH antagonist Nal-Glu in controlled ovarian hyperstimulation. *Fertil Steril* 1991;56:923–7
16. Olivennes F, Fanchin R, Bouchard P, *et al*. The single or dual administration of the gonadotrophin-releasing hormone antagonist cetrorelix in an *in vitro* fertilization–embryo transfer programme. *Fertil Steril* 1994;62:468–76

17. Leroy I, d'Acremont MF, Brailly-Tabard S, et al. A single injection of gonadotropin-releasing hormone (GnRH) antagonist (cetrorelix) postpones the luteinizing hormone (LH) surge: further evidence for the role of GnRH during the LH-surge. *Fertil Steril* 1997;62:461–7
18. Cassidenti DL, Sauer MV, Paulson RJ, et al. Comparison of intermittent and continuous use of a gonadotropin-releasing hormone antagonist (Nal-Glu) in *in vitro* fertilization cycles: a preliminary report. *Am J Obstet Gynecol* 1991;165:1806–10
19. Minaretzis D, Alper MM, Oskowitz SP, Lobel SM, Mortola JF, Pavlou SN. Gonadotropin-releasing hormone antagonist versus agonist administration in women undergoing controlled ovarian hyperstimulation: cycle performance and *in vitro* steroidogenesis of granulosa–lutein cells. *Am J Obstet Gynecol* 1994;172:1518–25
20. Felberbaum R, Reissmann T, Küpker W, et al. Hormone profiles under ovarian stimulation with human menopausal gonadotrophin (hMG) and concomitant administration of the gonadotrophin releasing hormone (GnRH)-antagonist cetrorelix at different dosages. *J Assist Reprod Gen* 1996;13:216–22
21. Albano C, Smitz J, Camus M, et al. Hormonal profile during the follicular phase in cycles stimulated with a combination of human menopausal gonadotrophin and gonadotrophin-releasing hormone antagonist (cetrorelix). *Hum Reprod* 1996;11:2114–18
22. Albano C, Smitz J, Camus M, Riethmüller-Winzen H, Van Steirteghem A, Devroey P. Comparison of different doses of gonadotropin-releasing hormone antagonist cetrorelix during controlled ovarian hyperstimulation. *Fertil Steril* 1997;67:917–22
23. Olivennes F, Fanchin R, Bouchard P, Taieb J, Selva J, Frydman R. Scheduled administration of a gonadotrophin-releasing hormone antagonist (cetrorelix) on day 8 of *in-vitro* fertilization cycles: a pilot study. *Hum Reprod* 1995;10:1382–6
24. Adashi EY. Endocrinology of the ovary. *Hum Reprod* 1994;9(Suppl 2):36–51
25. Schoot DC, Harlin J, Shoham Z, et al. Recombinant human follicle-stimulating hormone and ovarian response in gonadotrophin-deficient women. *Hum Reprod* 1994;9:1237–42
26. The Ganirelix Dose-finding Study Group. A double-blind, randomized, dose finding study to assess the efficacy of the gonadotrophin-releasing hormone antagonist ganirelix (Org 37462) to prevent premature luteinizing hormone surges in women undergoing ovarian stimulation with recombinant follicle stimulating hormone (Puregon®). *Hum Reprod* 1998;13:3023–31
27. Spona J, Coy DH, Zatlasch E, Wakolbinger C. LHRH antagonist inhibits gonadal steroid secretion *in vitro*. *Peptides* 1985;6:379–82
28. Srivastava RK, Sridaran R. Inhibition of luteal steroidogenesis by two LHRH antagonists (Nal-Glu and Nal-Arg antagonists) in the pregnant rat. *Endocr Res* 1994;20:365–76
29. Rongières-Bertrand C, Olivennes F, Righini C, et al. Revival of the natural cycles in *in-vitro* fertilization with the use of a new gonadotropin-releasing hormone antagonist (cetrorelix): a pilot study with minimal stimulation. *Hum Reprod* 1999;14:683–8

BIBLIOGRAPHY

Abstracts of relevant papers presented at the 5th International Symposium on GnRH Analogues in Cancer and Human Reproduction

24. Introduction to the GnRH antagonist ganirelix (Orgalutran®). B. Mannaerts, J. Oberyé, M. Peters, E. Orlemans, The Netherlands
26. Clinical outcome of a multi-centre trial of ganirelix (Orgalutran®) in women undergoing controlled ovarian hyperstimulation. B. Tarlatzis, B. Mannaerts, Greece, The Netherlands
27. Comparison in a prospective multicentric randomized study in IVF-ET of a single dose of GnRH antagonist (Cetrorelix) to a GnRH agonist long protocol (Triptoreline in depot formula). F. Olivennes, J. Belaisch-Allart, J.C. Emperaire, *et al.*, France
28. Cetrorelix in controlled ovarian stimulation for ART: results of phase III, multiple dose treatment. R.E. Felberbaum, Germany
29. Potential benefits of GnRH-antagonists in assisted reproduction. R.F. Casper, Canada
30. Cetrorelix levels in plasma and follicular fluid. M. Ludwig, R. Felberbaum, C. Albano, *et al.*, Germany, Belgium, France
31. New concepts in COS-ART related to the use of LHRH antagonists. P. Devroey, C. Albano, J. Smitz, R. Felberbaum, K. Diedrich, Germany
37. Ganirelix (Orgalutran®) in controlled ovarian stimulation before IVF/ICSI. T. Hillensjö, K. Borg, A.S. Forsberg, M. Wikland, M. Wood, Sweden
100. Safety aspects of GnRH antagonists. H. Riethmüller-Winzen, M. Siebert-Weigel, A. Prothmann, Germany
101. Effects of GnRH-agonist and antagonists on steroid production in rat and human granulosa cells. P.M. Verbost, J. Smitz, C. Peddemors, R. van de Lagemaat, H.J. Kloosterboer, P. Devroey, The Netherlands, Belgium

4
Application of GnRH analogues in the management of female infertility

E. Lunenfeld

Ever since the isolation, structural elucidation and synthesis of porcine gonadotropin hormone releasing hormone (GnRH), pGlu1-His2-Trp3-Ser4-Tyr5-Gly6-Leu7-Arg8-Pro9-Gly10NH$_2$, by Schally and co-workers[1], the interest in the application of GnRH analogues has experienced an explosive growth rate. It prompted intensive activities in the field of chemical synthesis and pharmacology of GnRH analogues by many laboratories.

The potency of GnRH and its analogues as stimulators, when administered in a precise pulsatile fashion, or inhibitors of pituitary gonadotropin secretion, when administered chronically, permitted its use as an ovulation inducer on the one hand, and as a method of 'reversible medical gonadectomy' applied to treatment of gonadal steroid-dependent diseases on the other hand. However, the usefulness of GnRH for use as an ovulation inducer or as a method of 'reversible medical gonadectomy' was limited by its rapid metabolic degradation by endopeptidases in position 6 of the molecule and consequently short half-life of about 2–5 min. Therefore, the primary chemical goals were to stabilize the molecule against enzymatic degradation and to increase the duration of action. Modifications of the molecule in positions 6 and 10 led to more stable compounds with higher potency and a half-life in humans of about 2–3 h after one single injection of 1 mg.

The effort invested in chemical synthesis during the early 1970s culminated with the discovery of several very potent agonists. Six of them are currently approved drugs (Figure 1). All the GnRH agonists contain a D-amino acid at position 6, which buttresses the peptide against enzymatic degradation and increases its receptor binding affinity by stabilizing the bioactive conformation. The agonists leuprolide, buserelin, goserelin and histrelin are nonapeptides and contain either

Table 1 GnRH agonists available as approved drugs

Name	Structure	Route of administration
Leuprolide	pGlu-His-Trp-Ser-Tyr-DLeu-Leu-Arg-Pro-NHEt	sc, depot, 2- and 3-month depot
Buserelin	pGlu-His-Trp-Ser-Tyr-DSer(O'Bu)-Leu-Arg-Pro-NHEt	sc, nasal, depot, 3-month depot
Nafarelin	pGlu-His-Trp-Ser-Tyr-D2Nal-Leu-Arg-Pro-GlyNH$_2$	sc, nasal
Goserelin	pGlu-His-Trp-Ser-Tyr-DScr(O'Bu)-Leu-Arg-Pro-AzaglyNH$_2$	sc, depot
Histrelin	pGlu-His-Trp-Ser-Tyr-DHis(Bzl)-Leu-Arg-Pro-AzaglyNH$_2$	sc
Triptorelin	pGlu-His-Trp-Ser-Tyr-DTrp-Leu-Arg-Pro-GlyNH$_2$	sc, depot

sc, subcutaneous

ethylamide or Azagly at position 10 (Table 1). Nafarelin and triptorelin contain the original Gly^{10} amide and are therefore decapeptides.

Thus, the structure of GnRH agonists is very similar to the native occurring GnRH. These GnRH agonists – as nonapeptides – were suitable for various hormone-dependent benign and malignant diseases, and they were first introduced in the market as a daily injection for the treatment of prostate cancer. In 1984, the use of the GnRH agonist buserelin, in association with human menopausal gonadotropin (hMG), was first reported for use in *in vitro* fertilization (IVF)[2]. The combined pituitary suppression/gonadotropin–ovarian stimulation therapy consists of two distinctive elements: pituitary suppression and ovarian stimulation. Each element exerts specific positive and adverse effects, and only the combination of all the corollaries produces the desired end result.

Application of a GnRH agonist leads to a rapid increase of gonadotropins, luteinizing hormone (LH), follicle stimulating hormone (FSH), and sexual steroids, such as estradiol in females and testosterone in males (flare-up), followed by a down-regulation of receptors, a desensitization, and consequently a suppression of both FSH and LH followed by suppression of sexual steroids to castration levels. The LH suppression was responsible for the prevention of premature LH surges. Premature luteinization dropped from 18 to 2% after treatment with GnRH agonists in assisted reproductive technology programs.

With time, various protocols were developed:

(1) Ultra-short protocol;

(2) Short (flare-up) protocol;

(3) Long protocol;

(4) Long protocol, e.g. with a preceding contraceptive cycle to prevent flare-up reaction and induce synchronization of oocyte development;

(5) Long-term down-regulation (ultra-long) protocol;

(6) Ovulation induction with GnRH agonist instead of an application of human chorionic gonadotropin (hCG) in clomiphene citrate cycles or in cycles stimulated by hMG without GnRH agonist pretreatment;

(7) Ovulation induction with GnRH agonist in cycles pretreated with GnRH antagonists;

(8) Screening/stimulation tests to predict optimum fertilization based on the rise of estradiol levels.

The ultra-short and short protocols make use of the initial stimulatory effect of gonadotropin secretion (flare-up) to promote follicular development before pituitary desensitization occurs. The GnRH agonist is usually given from cycle day 1, for 3 days in the ultra-short protocol or until injection of hCG in the short or flare-up protocol. Gonadotropin stimulation is started 2–3 days after initiation of the GnRH agonist administration. Some have recommended starting both the GnRH agonist and FSH on cycle day 3 when using the short protocol, in order to enhance follicular recruitment and growth. The short regimens have the advantage compared to the long protocol of having a shorter duration of stimulation, with fewer ampules of gonadotropins used and lower costs. There is no significant advantage in the precise timing of hCG injection after pituitary desensitization with the GnRH agonists, which has led to the notion that IVF therapy can be greatly simplified.

In the long protocols, the intent is to achieve pituitary down-regulation with suppression of endogenous gonadotropins, before stimulation with exogenous FSH. There are two regimens of the long protocol: the long follicular protocol involves the administration of GnRH agonist from cycle day 1 for approximately 12–14 days, whereas the long luteal protocol involves the administration of GnRH agonist from the mid-luteal phase of the previous cycle. For this purpose, the GnRH agonist is administered either daily or in the form of depot preparation from the mid-luteal or early follicular phase.

The timing of GnRH agonist administration during the menstrual cycle may influence the time course of ovarian suppression, but results in the literature are contradictory when mid-luteal and early follicular protocols are compared regarding time and effectiveness[3-5]. It seems, therefore, that the question is still open whether the GnRH agonist in long protocols should be started during the luteal phase of the preceding cycle or during the early follicular phase of the treatment cycle. At the present meeting, Tan [41] compared the GnRH agonist in long protocols starting at the early follicular phase to GnRH agonists following the use of combined oral contraceptive pills for 14 days. He demonstrated that the use of combined oral contraceptive pills for 14 days prior to the use of GnRH reduces cyst formations and gonadotropin requirement as well as making logistics easier.

The use of long-protocol regimens was associated with both increased folliculogenesis and an improved endocrine milieu[6]. Regan and colleagues[7] demonstrated that an elevated LH serum level was associated with a significant impairment of fertility and a notable increase in the rate of miscarriage. Furthermore, studies have shown that, in patients with polycystic ovary (PCO) syndrome, those having infertility problems have significantly higher LH concentrations than those who do not[8]. With the long protocol, LH can be profoundly suppressed and the miscarriage rate is significantly reduced. Similar findings were reported by Dodson and colleagues[9] who found a significant decrease of serum LH, estradiol and testosterone after a daily injection of leuprorelin acetate for 4 weeks, but no decrease of serum progesterone, FSH and dehydroepiandrosterone in patients with PCO syndrome. Compared to ovulation induction using hMG alone, leuprorelin acetate administration before and during hMG treatment prevented preovulatory rises in serum LH and progesterone concentrations. The authors concluded that the leuprorelin acetate administered to women with PCO syndrome decreases gonadal steroid production and is capable of preventing premature luteinization during ovulation induction with hMG.

Johnson and Pearce[10] confirmed that, in women with PCO syndrome and recurrent spontaneous abortions, pituitary suppression with GnRH analogues before induction of ovulation significantly reduced the increased spontaneous abortion rate.

In infertility caused by all stages of endometriosis, GnRH agonist treatment for 3 months, prior to ovarian stimulation, gave the highest fertilization rate. The embryo transfer rate was higher in GnRH agonist-pretreated patients than in patients treated with clomiphene citrate–hMG[11].

Marcus and Edwards[12] obtained similar results in patients with severe endometriosis. Down-regulation for 4 months increased pregnancy rates from 12.7% in controls to 42.8% in the GnRH agonist-treated patients. The superiority of the long protocol over the short protocol was confirmed by extensive meta-analysis[13].

Situation analysis demonstrated that, to date, about 85% of treatment cycles use the combination of gonadotropins + GnRH agonists. This has improved pregnancy rates, compared to 'non-agonists cycles' and has allowed programming and convenient timing for oocyte recovery. However, the use of GnRH agonists in the long protocol increased the treatment time, the amount of gonadotropins and the cost for each treatment cycle. Moreover, the use of the long protocol necessitated luteal support.

For stimulation, GnRH agonists can be combined with hMG as well as with FSH. The total consumption of gonadotropin ampules and the necessary days for stimulation depend on the galenical formulation and dose of the GnRH agonists and whether they are used as daily injections or depot formulations[14].

The main issues in the application of GnRH analogues in the management of female infertility discussed during the present meeting were the presentations of the results of phase III clinical trials using the novel GnRH antagonists (cetrorelix and ganirelix), comparing them to the well-established long protocols using GnRH agonists (buserelin and triptorelin) [26, 27, 28, 37].

GnRH antagonists cause a faster and more pronounced LH suppression. Early ovarian hyperstimulation syndrome might be prevented in protocols using a GnRH antagonist by using recombinant LH or GnRH agonist instead of hCG for ovulation induction [30]. Long-acting GnRH agonists should therefore be preferred to short-acting antagonists in indications where a longer suppression of sexual hormone production before controlled ovarian hyperstimulation is necessary, as is the case, for example, in endometriosis and in PCO syndrome as long as long-acting GnRH antagonists will not be available. Furthermore, all protocols using the benefit of flare-up reaction are uniquely reserved to GnRH agonists. The short treatment course with GnRH antagonists is appreciated by the patients.

In all studies with the antagonists, the duration of stimulation was shorter, and the amount of gonadotropins lower. However, this coincided with a trend of fewer follicles and oocytes as well as lower estrogens. Nevertheless, oocyte and embryo qualities were similar. Moreover, although the mean numbers of embryos transferred were equal, a consistent reduction in clinical pregnancy rate has been observed among the patients who received the antagonist in comparison to those who received the agonists. The lower pregnancy rate observed in the group of patients who received the antagonists coincided with a lower moderate and severe hyperstimulation syndrome. The reasons for this unexpected outcome have to be explored. The possible explanation of this phenomenon must be related to the interaction between embryo and endometrium. This may be due to direct effects of GnRH antagonists on the endometrium, or through reduction of LH and/or LH-induced angiogenic factors such as vascular endothelial growth factor (VEGF). Table 2 indicates possible preferences for GnRH agonist or GnRH antagonist in various protocols. For depot GnRH antagonists, the positioning can only be speculative due to a lack of data.

Table 2 GnRH agonist versus antagonist

Protocols/indications	Agonist daily s.c.	Agonist depot	Antagonist daily s.c.	Antagonist depot
Prevention of mid-cycle LH surge	+++	+++	+++	+++
Ultra-short protocol (use of flare-up reaction)	++	Ø	Ø	Ø
Short protocol (use of flare-up reaction)	++	Ø	Ø	Ø
Long protocol	++	+++	Ø	+++
Ultra-long protocol (PCO, fibroma, endometriosis)	+	+++	Ø	+++
Quality of oocytes/embryos	+++	+++	+++	NA
Pregnancy rate	+++	+++	++	NA
Carry-over effect (requirement of luteal phase support)	– –	– – –	–	–
Amount of gonadotropin ampules	– –	– – –	+	NA
Dose-dependent effect	++	++	–	–
Immediate LH suppression	–	–	+++	+++
Flare-up reaction	– –	– –	+++	+++
Screening/stimulation test (prediction of fertilization based on estradiol serum levels)	+++	Ø	Ø	Ø

+, advantages; – disadvantages; Ø, not applicable; NA, not available; s.c., subcutaneous; PCO, polycystic ovary syndrome

Currently, the only benefit of GnRH antagonists in the field of assisted reproduction seems to be prevention of a premature LH surge. This is also possible with GnRH agonists, with a decrease from 18 to 2%. However, preliminary data indicate that GnRH antagonists reduce the premature LH surge to a more pronounced extent (< 2%) and seem to necessitate a shorter treatment time and less medication. Furthermore, since GnRH antagonists cause a faster LH suppression, they may be administered later during the treatment and for a shorter period of time.

CONCLUSION

The introduction of GnRH analogues into protocols for assisted reproductive technologies was an exciting development in the control of follicular stimulation. The increased number of oocytes and embryos, and improved pregnancy rates, far outweight the requirement of additional medication and increased gonadotropin dose. They are safe and valuable pharmaceutical tools in the management of ovarian stimulation; it is yet too early to speculate about the possible end of the agonist era.

REFERENCES

1. Schally AV, Arimura A, Bowers CY, et al. Hypothalamic neurohormones regulating anterior pituitary function. *Rec Progr Horm Res* 1968;24:497
2. Porter RN, Smith W, Craft IL, et al. Induction of ovulation for *in vitro* fertilization using buserelin and gonadotropins. *Lancet* 1984;II:1284–5
3. Meldrum DR, Wilot A, Hamilton S, et al. Timing of initiation and dose schedule of leuprolide influence the time course of ovarian suppression. *Fertil Steril* 1988;50:400–7
4. Pellicier A, Simon C, Miro F, et al. Ovarian response and outcome of *in vitro* fertilization in patients treated with gonadotropin releasing analogue in different phases of the menstrual cycle. *Hum Reprod* 1989;4:285–9
5. Ron-El R, Herman A, Golan A, et al. The comparison of early and mid luteal administration of long acting gonadotropin releasing hormone agonist. *Fertil Steril* 1990;54:233–7
6. Filicori M, Cognigni GE, Arnone A, et al. Endocrine and clinical characteristics of different GnRH agonist regimens used for gonadotropin ovulation induction. In Filicori M, Flamigni C, eds. *Treatment with GnRH Analogs*. Proceedings of a Satellite Symposium of the 15th World Congress on Fertility and Sterility, Bologna, Italy, 15–16 September 1995, Chapter 22:183–7
7. Regan L, Owen EJ, Jacobs HS. Hypersecretion of luteinising hormone, infertility and miscarriage. *Lancet* 1990;336:1141–4
8. Conway GS, Honour JW, Jacobs HS. Heterogenicity of the polycystic ovary syndrome: clinical, endocrine and ultrasound features in 556 patients. *Clin Endocrinol* 1989;30:459–70
9. Dodson WC, Hughes CL, et al. The effect of leuprolide acetate on ovulation induction with human menopausal gonadotropins in polycystic ovary syndrome. *J Clin Endocrinol Metab* 1987;65:95–100
10. Johnson P, Pearce JM. Recurrent spontaneous abortion and polycystic ovarian disease: comparison of two regimens to induce ovulation. *Br Med J* 1995;311:231

11. Chedid S, Camus M, Smitz J, Van Steirteghem AC, Devroey P. Comparison among different ovarian stimulation regimens for assisted procreation procedures in patients with endometriosis. *Hum Reprod* 1995;10:2406–11
12. Marcus SF, Edwards RG. High rates of pregnancy after long-term down-regulation of women with severe endometriosis. *Am J Obstet Gynecol* 1994;171:812–17
13. Daya S. Optimal protocol for gonadotropin releasing hormone agonist use in ovarian stimulation. In Gomel V, Cheung PCK, eds. *In Vitro Fertilization and Assisted Reproduction.* Bologna: Monduzzi Editore, 1997:405–15
14. Fabregues F, Balasch J, *et al.* Long-term down-regulation does not improve pregnancy rates in an *in vitro* fertilization program. *Fertil Steril* 1998;70:46–51

BIBLIOGRAPHY

Abstracts of relevant papers presented at the 5th International Symposium on GnRH Analogues in Cancer and Human Reproduction

26. Clinical outcome of a multicentre trial of ganirelix (Orgalutran®) in women undergoing controlled ovarian hyperstimulation. B. Tarlatzis, B. Mannaerts, The Netherlands
27. Comparison in a prospective multicentric randomized study in IVF-ET of a single dose of GnRH antagonist (cetrorelix) to a GnRH agonist long protocol (triptorelin) in depot formula. F. Olivennes, J. Belaisch-Allart, J.C. Emperaire, B. Hedon, S. Alvarez, L. Moreau, B. Nicollet, J.R. Zorn, P. Bouchard, R. Frydman, France
28. Cetrorelix in controlled ovarian stimulation for ART: results of phase III multiple dose treatment. R.E. Felberbaum, Germany
30. Cetrorelix levels in plasma and follicular fluid. M. Ludwig, R. Felberbaum, C. Albano, F. Olivennes, H. Riethmüller-Winzen, P. Devroey, K. Diedrich, Germany and France
37. Ganirelix (Orgalutran®) in controlled ovarian stimulation before IVF/ICSI. T. Hillensjö, K. Borg, A.S. Forsberg, M. Wikland, M. Wood, Sweden
41. Use of oral contraceptive and LHRH agonist for patients scheduling in ART. S.L. Tan, Canada

5
GnRH analogues: safety aspects
K. Bühler

INTRODUCTION

In the past two decades, the impact of gonadotropin releasing hormone (GnRH) analogues (GnRHa) on the management of many sex hormone-dependent pathologies has become evident. In the very beginning of the clinical use of this compound, only a few indications for its use could be imagined, so it is all the more fascinating to see in how many fields of endocrinological therapy the use of GnRH agonists has become routine today. At the end of this century and millennium the first GnRH antagonists will be introduced on the market.

From the use of GnRH agonists over the past two decades we learned much about the physiology and pathophysiology of the GnRH effects and metabolism. With our large experience in this field we are able to emphasize that GnRH agonists have been proved to be efficient drugs. However, it is not only efficacy that must be studied very carefully but also safety aspects, especially when such drugs are used in large amounts in the field of human reproduction.

GENERAL SIDE-EFFECTS

It is interesting that all the reported side-effects from GnRH agonists depend strongly on the estradiol deprivation caused by agonists and not on a direct effect of the drug[1]. First experiences with the chronic application of an antagonist depot formulation, abarelix depot [103], in endometriosis also showed no clinical adverse events attributable directly to the drug. Owing to prolonged hormonal treatment with GnRH agonists (for example for endometriosis, uterine fibroids, metastatic breast cancer or *in vitro* fertilization (IVF)), metabolic, endocrine, hemostatic or psychological disturbances had to be excluded. No negative influences during agonist treatment could be found on general metabolic parameters such as electrolyte balance, white blood cell count, platelet and hemoglobin levels, liver, kidney and lipid metabolism or atherogenic index [96]. A positive effect was demonstrated on hemostasis: agonist pretreatment appeared to be beneficial in avoiding thromboembolic complications, particularly in those patients undergoing surgery or prolonged bedrest[2] and on hemoglobin levels in anemic patients prior to treatment.

It is understandable that symptoms depending on estradiol were not seen when GnRH antagonists were used in patients undergoing controlled ovarian hyperstimulation (COH), owing to the short duration of application. The antagonist was administered in a single dose of 3 mg or as a multiple dose of 0.25 mg daily for several days. Side-effects were injection-site reactions reported by 1.6% (0.25 mg doses) and 20.6% (3 mg cetrorelix) [100] and 17.1% (ganirelix 0.25 mg) of treated patients [24], nausea (0.5%) and headache (0.2%) [100].

BONE MINERAL DENSITY AND ADD-BACK THERAPY

In past years the concomitant symptoms caused by the extreme decrease of estradiol during the chronic application of GnRHa gave rise to the so-called add-back therapy. The aim of this add-back therapy is two-fold. On the one hand, it aims to avoid extreme bone loss as a consequence of the decrease in estradiol experienced in the postmenopausal state of a woman. A 6-month course of GnRH agonist therapy causes an average decrease in bone mineral density of 2–6%. These changes are significant but remain within the normal age-specific ranges. After cessation of GnRH agonist treatment, there is a complete or at least a partial restoration of bone mineral density[3].

On the other hand, add-back therapy is used to decrease intolerable side-effects such as hot flushes, sweating, sleep disturbances and others. The therapeutic effect, however, should not be negatively influenced by the add-back therapy. Hornstein and co-workers[4] showed, in a randomized, placebo-controlled comparative study, that, with higher dosages of estradiol with or without a combination with norethisterone, loss of bone mineral density can effectively be avoided, but with higher dosages there is also a significant decrease in reduction of endometriosis-related pain symptoms. Cedars and associates[5] showed that, in combination with 20–30 mg of medroxyprogesterone acetate, no significant reduction in rAFS scores could be achieved, over that with the GnRH agonist treatment alone. An alternative without a supplementary application of sex steroids might be, for example, repeated 3-month courses of GnRH agonist treatment, which significantly relieved recurrent endometriotic symptoms and signs without sustained loss of bone mineral density[6]. In case of uterine fibroma, following a conventional course of GnRH agonist, maintenance at a very low dose avoids both recurrence of uterine leiomyoma and bone mineral loss[7]. Other possibilities for additional treatment could be seen in biphosphonates for bone mineral density loss prevention[8,9] or in melatonin for prevention of insomnia[10].

CENTRAL PRECOCIOUS PUBERTY AND MALIGNANT DISEASES

In children with central precocious puberty (CPP), the administration of GnRH agonists even over years has few side-effects [99]. Symptoms that could suggest an anaphylactic or anaphylactoid reaction have been very rare. To date no long-term side-effects have been observed. Two years after discontinuing therapy, lumbar and hip bone mineral density were normal for skeletal age. Normal function of the pituitary–ovary/testis axis was re-established. Hyperandrogenism and polycystic ovarian disease seen in girls treated for CPP have to be regarded as symptoms of CPP and not as a consequence of the GnRH agonist treatment. Histological changes seen in the testes of men treated with GnRH agonists for prostatic cancer[11] or in animal experiments in rats cannot be transferred to young boys treated for CPP[12]. No irreversible testicular damage in humans clearly deriving from GnRH agonist treatment has been described[13]. In young women undergoing chemotherapy for lymphoma and leukemia, GnRH agonist co-treatment was able to exert a protective effect on ovarian function [66]. The pseudo-prepubertal ovaries were more resistant to alkylating agents. Also, in the treatment of prostatic cancer, the GnRH agonist therapy provides better quality of life. Ludwig and colleagues [82] reported that men younger than 75 years suffered more from surgical orchiectomy than from GnRH agonist treatment.

FLARE-UP AND INADVERTENT PREGNANCY EXPOSURE

Sometimes the initiation of the agonist treatment can lead to so-called flare-up complications such as long-lasting and strong menstruation, cyst formation or rapid increase in the size of endometriomata. Prevention of such initial flare-up effects is possible by starting the GnRH agonist during pretreatment with an oral ethinylestradiol/progestagen combination (e.g. oral contraceptive), especially in cases of large ovarian endometriomata or before IVF treatment[12,14]. Other beneficial effects could be seen with this combination therapy: pituitary suppression was achieved more rapidly and there was a clear reduction of the risk of administering the agonist inadvertently in an unnoticed pregnancy or of allowing conception during the flare-up phase[15]. A flare-up effect is not seen when the GnRH antagonist is initiated [100, 103, 104]. With this compound a prompt and rapid reduction in serum levels of luteinizing hormone (LH), follicle stimulating hormone (FSH) and estradiol is achieved. Daya [98] reported an incidence of inadvertent GnRH agonist exposure in early pregnancy of 0.82%. In animal studies on the effect of GnRH agonist exposure, only a poor fetal outcome was reported. In humans to date, 422 exposed pregnancies have been reported. From 319 babies, data were available showing premature delivery in 19 cases and five babies small for dates. Five babies showed congenital anomalies (including bilateral talipes, cleft palate and hypospadias). The rest of the babies born at term were classified as normal. The data obtained from case reports and case series indicate that, in humans, the administration of a GnRH agonist in early pregnancy is not associated with an adverse outcome for the pregnancy. The recommendation for the management of the exposed pregnancy must consist of counselling, progesterone support, detailed ultrasonography and high-risk monitoring. Future investigations in this field have to clarify whether the risk depends on the type of protocol used and the role of inhibin proalpha C in predicting outcome. The risk of inadvertent exposure can be reduced by the simultaneous use of oral contraceptives as mentioned above. In all cases we need a registry for long-term follow-up.

Regarding the current protocols for the use of the antagonists in COH, it seems very unlikely that inadvertent injection into an ongoing pregnancy will occur. There are first reports of depot formulations of a GnRH antagonist for chronic application in endometriosis, such as abarelix depot [103], or in uterine fibroids, such as a depot formulation of cetrorelix [13]. From the cetrorelix slow-release formulation it is known that ovulations occurred during the treatment. With an increasing use of such antagonist depot preparations, there will be an increasing risk of inadvertent administration of the antagonist into an ongoing pregnancy.

EFFECT ON REPRODUCTIVE TISSUES

Another very important question in this context is whether GnRHa may be able to exert a direct unfavorable effect on the ovary, the oocyte, granulosa cells or the trophoblast itself. Dodson and co-workers[16] showed that serum, follicular and peritoneal fluid concentrations were undetectable 2 days after discontinuation of the GnRH agonist leuprolide (day from human chorionic gonadotropin (hCG) administration to oocyte retrieval). There was no measurable effect on granulosa–lutein cell progesterone accumulation *in vitro* nor on human or murine embryo growth rates up to the 8-cell stage *in vitro*. Verbost and colleagues [101] showed *in vitro* that, in human granulosa luteal cells – and probably in preovulatory granulosa cells also, neither GnRH agonists nor GnRH antagonists had any effect on sex steroid secretion in the presence or absence of hCG. Ortmann and co-workers [102] tested the

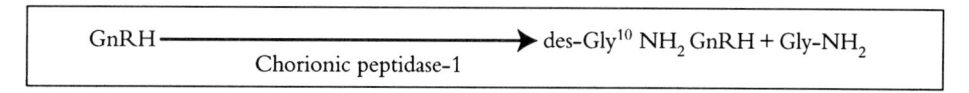

$$\text{GnRH} \xrightarrow[\text{Chorionic peptidase-1}]{} \text{des-Gly}^{10}\text{ NH}_2\text{ GnRH + Gly-NH}_2$$

Figure 1 Action of chorionic peptidase-1

effect of GnRHa on cultured human granulosa cells obtained from patients treated in different protocols for COH receiving triptorelin (agonist), cetrorelix or ganirelix (antagonist) or no GnRHa. Such *in vivo* treatment also did not result in significant actions of the GnRHa on spontaneous or hCG-stimulated steroidogenesis.

It is not only the effect of GnRHa on granulosa cells that has to be studied, however. GnRH also plays an important role during early pregnancy, being synthesized by and having biological effects on the human placenta [97]. Lin and co-workers[17] reported the expression of a human GnRH receptor gene in the placenta. Related to gestational age, GnRH stimulates hCG secretion by the trophoblast[18-20]. However, in pregnant women in whom the maternal circulation showed a pathological GnRH-binding substance, significantly lower levels of hCG were found. It must also be taken into consideration that there is a specific GnRH metabolism in the trophoblast. The placenta disposes of a very active enzymatic system, chorionic peptidase-1, which acts as a post-proline peptidase to degrade GnRH and which may protect it from exogenous GnRH and preserve the paracrine function of endogenous chorionic GnRH (Figure 1).

The placental content of this peptidase is notable and enough to inactivate 2350 fmol of GnRH per min[21]. Although the C-terminal ethylamide inhibition of the degradation of GnRH agonists is approximately ten-fold that of genuine analogues of GnRH, agonists as well as antagonists, which are not altered at position 9, are also degraded by chorionic peptidase-1. Thus, in pregnancy, the GnRH agonists do not act as superagonists in the intrauterine tissues, as they do at the pituitary, probably owing to their rapid degradation by chorionic peptidase-1[22]. In addition, since the chorionic receptor may differ from that of the pituitary, it may be possible to design new tailored analogues with little extrapituitary effect, for example on the endometrium, trophoblast, placenta and the embryo itself, preserving the activity in the pituitary.

ASSISTED REPRODUCTION

These tailored drugs will be very important in the future. Regarding the published results of comparative studies between agonists and antagonists in assisted reproduction, it becomes evident that, in pregnancy rates, there is a real difference between

Table 1 Pregnancy rates in several randomized studies comparing various GnRH antagonists with reference agonists

Abstract	GnRH antagonist	Dosage	Change in pregnancy rate (%)	GnRH agonist
26	ganirelix	0.25 mg daily	−5.7	buserelin
28	cetrorelix	0.25 mg daily	−7.0	buserelin
27	cetrorelix	3 mg once (twice)	−7.0	triptorelin (3.75 mg)

both drug classes [26, 27, 28] (Table 1). Even if in the particular study alone no significant difference could be found, in a meta-analysis of all these studies the statistical significance concerning pregnancy rates is evident (S. Daya, personal communication). Overall, significantly lower implantation and pregnancy rates were observed, although there were reported a similar number of oocytes collected, fertilization rates, number of oocytes transferred and oocyte and embryo quality in all the studies. Coelingh Bennink concluded that there must still exist an unknown class-related effect [104]. This effect on pregnancy rates seems to be dose dependent. In the ganirelix dose-finding study, there was a dramatic decrease in pregnancy rates and an extraordinary increase in early miscarriage rates when daily doses of 0.5 mg were used[23]. An important benefit from the use of antagonists could be seen in the fact that all studies reported a lower incidence of severe ovarian hyperstimulation syndrome (OHSS), probably related to the smaller (buserelin daily) or greater (triptorelin depot) increase in the need of gonadotropin for adequate follicle stimulation when agonists were used. In this context, it may also be of advantage that induction of meiosis can be performed in antagonist-treated patients without hCG but with GnRH or GnRH agonists. In a short time, recombinant LH will be available and, in the future, completely different principles might be introduced such as a meiosis-activating sterol[24].

SUMMARY AND FUTURE PERSPECTIVES

As has been known for nearly two decades, GnRH agonists produce few side-effects in clinical use. Larger experience with the administration of different GnRH antagonists has provided similar results. Concomitant symptoms, such as hot flushes, sweating, sleep disturbances and bone mineral density reduction depend on the degree and duration of GnRH analogue treatment, and are caused by estradiol deprivation. If these concomitant symptoms have too negative an influence on the patient's quality of life, add-back therapy is required. The principle of add-back therapy is that it should not interfere with the therapeutic aim. The initiation of agonist treatment together with an oral contraceptive provides two important benefits: prevention of flare-up complications and prevention of an accidental administration into an ongoing pregnancy. Even if the latter occurs, with all our experience today we can suggest that GnRH agonists have no deleterious effects on embryo viability and on the well-being of the fetus and the child. Future investigations must show that GnRH antagonists also, with their completely different mode of action and different metabolism with a higher amount of unnatural amino acids, exert no noxious effects. When antagonists are also used for long-term application in women of reproductive age, the risk of inadvertent exposure will become a reality.

The lower results in pregnancy rates require studies of the embryo–endometrium interaction and possible influences of agonists and antagonists. It is obvious that, with higher doses of antagonist during a follicle stimulation protocol, only lower pregnancy rates could be achieved. This is not because of an effect on the oocyte itself. With cryopreserved pronuclear-oocytes collected in treatment cycles with high GnRH antagonist doses, similar pregnancy rates were achieved compared with oocytes from low-dose treatment cycles. A direct effect of the antagonist cannot be excluded for the moment. We know that the embryo as well as the endometrium expresses the GnRH receptor[25]. Even if today we do not know the significance of such receptor expression, negative influences of the analogues must be excluded. The antagonist Nal-Glu completely blocked the GnRH-dependent dose–response effect of hCG secretion in placenta explant culture systems[17]. In the same way, the metabolism of the analogues needs further investigation. If, owing to the replacement of the genuine amino acid at position 10 by a C-terminal ethylamide, the molecular degradation by the peptidases is strongly inhibited, what will be the effect of replacing a completely different amino acid? With the introduction of these fascinating compounds on the market, we need answers in the interests of our patients.

GnRH agonists and GnRH antagonists have proved highly efficacious in the treatment of sex hormone-dependent diseases and in assisted reproduction. Considering all their enormous potential, only a few side-effects have been found and no really harmful disturbances have been described to date. We therefore look forward to developments in the next millennium.

REFERENCES

1. Bühler K. GnRH agonists and safety. In Lunenfeld B, Insler V, eds. *GnRH Analogues: The State of the Art 1993*. Carnforth, UK: Parthenon Publishing, 1993

2. Winkler U, Bühler K, Koslowski S, Oberhoff C, Schindler AE. Plasmatic haemostasis in gonadotrophin-releasing hormone analogue therapy: effects of leuprorelin acetate depot on coagulatory and fibrinolytic activities. *Clin Therapeut* 1992;14(Suppl a):114
3. Christiansen C, Christensen MS, Rodbro P, Hagen C, Transbol I. Effect of 1,25-dihydroxy-vitamin D_3 in itself or combined with hormone treatment in preventing postmenopausal osteoporosis. *Eur J Clin Invest* 1981;11:305–9
4. Hornstein MD, Surrey ES, Weisberg GW, Casino LA. Leuprolide acetate depot and hormonal add-back in endometriosis: a 12-month study. *Obstet Gynecol* 1998;91:16–24
5. Cedars MI, Lu JKH, Meldrum DR, Judd HL. Treatment of endometriosis with a long-acting gonadotropin-releasing hormone agonist plus medroxy-progesterone acetate. *Obstet Gynecol* 1990;75:641–5
6. Adamson GD, Heinrichs WL, Henzl MR, et al. Therapeutic efficacy and bone mineral density response during and following a three-month re-treatment of endometriosis with nafarelin (Synarel). *Am J Obstet Gynecol* 1997;177:1413–18
7. Broekmans FJ, Hompes PGA, Heitbrink MA, et al. Two-step gonadotropin-releasing hormone agonist treatment of uterine leiomyomas: standard-dose therapy followed by reduced-dose therapy. *Am J Obstet Gynecol* 1996; 175:1208–16
8. Herd RJ, Balena R, Blake GM, Ryan PJ, Fogelman I. The prevention of early postmenopausal bone loss by cyclical etidronate therapy: a 2-year, double-blind, placebo-controlled study. *Am J Med Aug* 1997;103:92–9
9. Surrey ES, Voigt B, Fournet N, Judd HL. Prolonged gonadotropin-releasing hormone agonist treatment of symptomatic endometriosis: the role of cyclic sodium etidronate and low-dose norethindrone 'add-back' therapy. *Fertil Steril* 1995;63:747–54
10. Amstrong SM. Melatonin as a chronbiotic for circadian insomnias: animal models and clinical observations. *Hanseatic Endocrine Conference: Melatonin after Four Decades: An Assessment of its Potential.* Hamburg, 1998
11. Waxman J, Lowe D, Whitfield HN, Hendry BF, Besser GM. The effects of a gonadotropin-releasing hormone agonist on testicular histology. *Fertil Steril* 1987;48:1067–9
12. Bühler K. The use of GnRH analogues in reproductive medicine. B. Safety aspects. *10th World Congress on In Vitro Fertilization and Assisted Reproduction.* Vancouver, 1996
13. Weinbauer GF, Nieschlag E. Reversibility of GnRH agonist-induced inhibition of testicular function: differences between rats and primates. *Prog Clin Biol Res* 1989;303: 75–87
14. Biljan MM, Mahutte NG, Dean N, Hemmings R, Bisonette F, Tan SL. Effects of pretreatment with an oral contraceptive on the time required to achieve pituitary suppression with gonadotrophin-releasing hormone analogues and on subsequent implantation and pregnancy rates. *Fertil Steril* 1998;70:1063–9
15. Bühler K. GnRH analogues: safety aspects. In Lunenfeld B, Insler V, eds. *GnRH Analogues: the State of the Art 1996.* Carnforth, UK: Parthenon Publishing, 1996
16. Dodson WC, Myers T, Morton PC, Conn PM. Leuprolide acetate: serum and follicular fluid concentrations and effects on human fertilization, embryo growth, and granulosa-lutein cell progesterone accumulation *in vitro. Fertil Steril* 1988;50:612–17
17. Lin LS, Roberts VJ, Yen SS. Expression of human gonadotropin-releasing hormone receptor gene in the placenta and its functional relationship to human chorionic gonadotropin secretion. *J Clin Endocrinol Metab* 1995;80:580–5
18. Gohar J, Mazor M, Leiberman JR. GnRH in pregnancy. *Arch Gynecol Obstet* 1996;259:1–6

19. Iwashita M, Kudo Y, Shinozaki Y, Takeda Y. Gonadotropin-releasing hormone increases serum human chorionic gonadotropin in pregnant women. *Endocr J* 1993;40:539–44
20. Szilagyi A, Benz R, Rossmanith WG. The human first-term placenta *in vitro*: regulation of hCG secretion by GnRH and its antagonist. *Gynecol Endocrinol* 1992;6:293–300
21. Kang IS, Siler-Khodr TM. Chorionic peptidase inactivates GnRH as a postproline peptidase. *Placenta* 1992;13:81–7
22. Siler-Khodr TM, Kang IS, Kuehl TJ, Khodr GS. Potential for embryo damage by GnRH analogs. In Filicori M, Flamigni C, eds. *Ovulation Induction: Basis, Science and Clinical Advances*. Amsterdam: Elsevier Science, 1994
23. Ganirelix Dose-finding Study Group. A double blind, randomized, dose-finding study to assess the efficacy of the gonadotrophin-releasing hormone antagonist ganirelix (Org 37462) to prevent premature luteinizing hormone surges in women undergoing ovarian stimulation with recombinant follicle stimulating hormone (Puregon7). *Hum Reprod* 1998;13:3023–31
24. Grøndahl C, Ottesen JL, Lessl M, *et al*. Meiosis-activating sterol promotes resumption of meiosis in mouse oocytes cultured *in vitro* in contrast to related oxysterols. *Biol Reprod* 1998;58:1297–302
25. Casañ EM, Raga F, Polan ML. GnRH mRNA and protein expression in human preimplantation embryos. *Mol Hum Reprod* 1999;5:234–9

BIBLIOGRAPHY

Abstracts of relevant papers presented at the 5th International Symposium on GnRH Analogues in Cancer and Human Reproduction

13. Medical management of uterine fibroids: GnRH antagonists. R.E. Felberbaum, Germany
24. Introduction to the GnRH antagonist ganirelix (Orgalutran®). B. Mannaerts, J. Oberyé, M. Peters, E. Orlemans, The Netherlands
26. Clinical outcome of a multi-centre trial of ganirelix (Orgalutran®) in women undergoing controlled ovarian hyperstimulation. B. Tarlatzis, B. Mannaerts, Greece, The Netherlands
27. Comparison in a prospective multicentric randomized study in IVF-ET of a single dose of GnRH antagonist (cetrorelix) to a GnRH agonist long protocol (triptorelin in depot formula). F. Olivennes, J. Belaisch-Allart, J.C. Emperaire, *et al*., France
28. Cetrorelix in controlled ovarian stimulation for ART: results of phase III, multiple dose treatment. R.E. Felberbaum, Germany
66. Preservation of ovarian function in young women undergoing chemotherapy. Z. Blumenfeld, Israel
82. Quality of life under different modalities of androgen-deprivation in advanced prostate cancer. G. Ludwig, W. Ohlig, H.J. Berberich, M. Steiger, Germany
96. Safety aspects of the use of GnRH agonists in benign and malign indications. K. Bühler, Germany
97. GnRH agonist and the trophoblast and embryo. T.M. Siler-Khodr, USA
98. The outcome of gonadotropin releasing hormone agonist (GnRHa) administration in early pregnancy. S. Daya, Canada
99. Safety aspects with GnRH analogues in precocious puberty. P.A. Lee, USA

100. Safety aspects of GnRH antagonists. H. Riethmüller-Winzen, M. Siebert-Weigel, A. Prothmann, Germany
101. Effects of GnRH-agonist and antagonists on steroid production in rat and human granulosa cells. P.M. Verbost, J. Smitz, C. Peddemors, R. van de Lagemaat, J.J. Kloosterboer, P. Devroey, The Netherlands, Belgium
102. Ovarian effects of GnRH antagonists. O. Ortmann, J.M. Weiss, E.M. Gürke, K. Oltmanns, R. Felberbaum, K. Diedrich, Germany
103. Initial safety profile and hormonal dose–response characteristics of the pure GnRH antagonist, abarelix-depot, in women with endometriosis. P.M. Martha, M.E. Gray, M. Campion, *et al.*, USA
104. Review on the use of GnRH antagonists for the treatment of infertility. H.J.T. Coelingh Bennink, The Netherlands

6
Current status of medical treatment of sex offenders with GnRH analogues

D. Seifert

Prompted by a few sensational sexual offences against children, the subject of treatment for this group of offenders and the question of how effective such treatment measures are have been keenly debated, even a matter of controversy, in recent years in Germany. A similar debate has taken place in the USA[1]. In January 1998 the German legislature passed an amendment to the criminal law which resulted in the lengthening of custodial sentences for certain sexual offences. Psychiatry and psychology experts are to be consulted increasingly when dealing with these offenders, especially when it comes to release, in other words when assessing the possibility of reoffending. It was also decided that more treatment options should be created for this group. The problem is that the treatability of these disorders is limited. The empirical findings available to date indicate that only some of those affected can be reached with the treatment methods currently in use.

In recent years there have been occasional studies on the use of gonadotropin releasing hormone analogues (GnRHa) to treat sex offenders. A few general facts about this group and about the treatment methods used up to now are presented. Sex offenders are defined from the legal point of view, i.e. they must have committed a criminal offence against 'the sexual self-determination of other persons' or 'caused death in order to satisfy their sexual urge'. The elements of these offences are firmly set out in the German penal code.

By contrast, medical and psychiatric differentiation is complex. The background to these acts can have a diversity of causes. These may include, for instance, a development-related conflict situation, a sexually expressed act of aggression or – less commonly the case – a fixated sexual deviation. According to the international classification of mental diseases (ICD-10 or DSM IV), disorders in the area of sexuality come under the heading 'disorders of sexual preference' or 'paraphilia'[2,3]. The most commonly observed forms of paraphilia are pedophilia and exhibitionism. Far less common are sadistic perverted developments such as sadomasochism and sexually motivated killing. Even the term pedophilia is merely a collective term, covering a variety of personality developments with their individual conflict dynamics.

In terms of the incidence of these disorders, the following figures are worth noting: in Germany 4981 people were convicted of a sexual offence in 1996[4]. This figure has stayed virtually constant since the 1950s and so has not increased, contrary to differing reports. Around three-quarters of the total of 4500 sex offenders serving custodial sentences in Germany are in prison and a quarter are in special psychiatric units – in order to carry out what are called necessary forensic measures[5]. Hence a minority of these offenders are actually receiving psychiatric or psychotherapeutic treatment. The term 'sex offender' clearly does not represent a uniform group and the treatment methods used are correspondingly diverse.

TREATMENT METHODS OF SEX OFFENDERS

Methodologically there are three different forms of treatment:

(1) Surgical castration;

(2) Psychotherapy;

(3) Drug treatment.

Surgical castration

Based on the biological and mechanistic assumption that sexual behavior is largely controlled by hormonal influences, especially that of testosterone, people became convinced of the value of performing surgical castration. However, there have been increasing moves away from this method in recent years because of the ethical problems and the irreversible nature of the operations. Currently no more than six of these surgical castrations are performed annually in Germany[6].

Psychotherapy

At present psychotherapy is the most commonly used treatment method. An extensive meta-analysis proved the effectiveness of this form of therapy[7]. It seems that cognitive behavioral therapy measures, in particular, have the effect of preventing reoffending. However, it is worth remembering that the number of qualified psychotherapists has hitherto been far too small.

Drug treatment

From an effective drug treatment for these disorders we should expect, ideally, that:

(1) The deviant behavior and deviant fantasies should be suppressed;

(2) Normal sexual activity should largely be maintained;

(3) The side-effect profile should be minimized.

This last point is particularly important because sex offenders usually lack any primary motivation to be treated. They rarely go to the doctor because of the strain of their condition. Drug treatments can be divided into four substance groups.

The antiandrogens

The first clinical trial on using the antiandrogen cyproterone acetate (CPA) among this group of offenders was published in 1971[8]. Since then 'medical castration' has virtually superseded surgical castration. The mode of action of CPA is based on blocking the androgen receptors at the target organs. This form of treatment, referred to as 'hormonal castration', was initially welcomed with great hopes. However, this method has also been the subject of increasing criticism since 1994, when suspicions of a carcinogenic effect on the liver came under discussion. Several studies have described the therapeutic effect of antiandrogens[9,10]. Critically it must be noted that the distribution of the study population was mostly non-uniform, making it difficult to generalize from the results of the (few) follow-up studies. Also, the blood levels of testosterone did not fall regularly and to the same extent in all patients – on average to about 25% of the original blood level[11]. Furthermore, a few patients reported an increase in frequency of masturbation and sexual fantasies. There were frequent complaints of side-effects.

Selective serotonin reuptake inhibitors

Selective serotonin reuptake inhibitors (SSRIs), such as fluoxetine, fluvoxamine and clomipramine, belong to the group of antidepressants and are usually employed in the treatment of depression, states of anxiety and obsessive compulsive disorders. Since the early 1990s there have been occasional papers on the use of these drugs to treat paraphilias. Positive effects were particularly noticeable when depressive symptoms were present concurrently or when the deviant fantasies took the form of obsessive compulsive thoughts[12,13].

Other psychotropic drugs

A large number of other drugs have an influence on sexual arousal. The inhibitory effect of neuroleptics – a group of drugs mainly used to treat schizophrenic psychoses – has been known since the 1960s. However, apart from a few case reports, there have been no extensive studies on their use in paraphilias[13].

Hormonal substances with a specific antiandrogenic profile

Medroxyprogesterone acetate (MPA) is the hormonal agent that has principally been used for the treatment of deviant sexual behavior in the USA[14,15]. Early experience of using GnRHa has also been available for a few years, but there are only a few studies[16–23] (Table 1).

The existing studies are largely based on case reports. No controlled trials exist. A total of 41 patients were studied in these eight papers. There are considerable differences in methodology. For instance, the period of follow-up ranged from a few weeks to as much as 7 years. A few patients were also treated with antiandrogens alternately or in combination. For these reasons, the comparability of these articles is limited.

The first scientific report on the use of GnRHa (leuprolide acetate) in patients with paraphilia comes from 1985[16]. This was a reader's letter in a weekly medical newsletter aimed primarily at internal medicine specialists and general practitioners, so detailed information about previous history, therapeutic procedure and follow-up are lacking.

Table 1 Studies on the use of GnRHa

Authors	Patients (n)	GnRHa
Allolio et al. (1985)[16]	1	leuprorelin
Rousseau et al. (1990)[17]	1	triptorelin
Dickey (1992)[18]	1	leuprorelin
Marcus et al. (1993)[19]	1	leuprorelin
Cooper and Cernovsky (1994)[20]	1	leuprorelin
Thibaut et al. (1993 and 1996)[21,22]	6	triptorelin
Rösler and Witztum (1998)[23]	30	triptorelin

Thibaut and colleagues[21,22] reported on six patients aged between 15 and 39 whom they treated with 3.75 mg triptorelin intramuscularly monthly for a period of up to 36 months. The longest observation period was 7 years. Two subjects committed another sexual offence 8 and 10 weeks after stopping the medication, which the authors attributed to the treatment period being too short (12 and 24 months, respectively). In the case of the other four subjects, a marked reduction in their sexually deviant fantasies was also recorded after withdrawal of the medication (up to 4 years). Erectility through to intercourse with orgasm, but without ejaculation, was preserved.

The most extensive study on this subject to date was published 1 year ago in *The New England Journal of Medicine*. Rösler and Witztum treated 30 subjects (average age 32 years) with pedophilia ($n = 25$) or some other, combined sexual deviation[23]. They gave monthly intramuscular injections of 3.75 mg triptorelin for treatment periods ranging from 12 to a maximum of 42 months. Six subjects discontinued the treatment between months 8 and 10. Three of these six experienced intolerable side-effects and their treatment was therefore changed to the antiandrogen CPA (200 mg/day); two of these three patients were convicted of further sexual offences.

All the 24 subjects who took triptorelin for more than a year showed a significant decrease in deviant sexual fantasies and desires no later than 3–10 months after the start of treatment. Deviant behavior completely stagnated. Mental well-being overall was stabilized. 'Normal' sexual interest declined, erectility was reduced, but possible, in the majority of subjects.

We have been treating sex offenders with leuprolide acetate for 1 year at our institute of forensic psychiatry. Our experience of the effect has been that it is comparable to the results of those studies already listed. For example, a 26-year-old man who had been sentenced to prison because of attempted manslaughter of a 9-year-old girl in order to satisfy his sexual urge was treated unsuccessfully with CPA. For the past 10 months we have given 37.5 mg leuprolide acetate intramuscularly, monthly. During the first 3 months the patient did not notice any change. From the 4th month on he has described a decrease in deviant fantasies and even seems to be more interested in psychotherapy. We must wait and see how things develop.

CONCLUSIONS

Despite the methodological limitation that no controlled trial on the treatment of paraphilia with GnRHa has yet been performed, the following points can be made based on the studies already referred to:

(1) GnRHa clearly exert an inhibitory effect on sexually deviant fantasies and acts. This seems remarkable in that more than half of the study subjects had previously been treated unsuccessfully with antiandrogens.

(2) The capacity for a 'normal' sex life seems to be reduced but entirely possible.

(3) There is agreement that concurrent psychotherapy should take place.

(4) The side-effect profile seems to be smaller than with the previously used alternatives CPA and MPA.

(5) The monthly depot injection is advantageous.

To summarize, interest in drug treatment for forms of paraphilia has grown in recent years. Overall the available findings indicate that GnRHa may play a significant role in the treatment of patients with paraphilia. They appear to meet the three conditions previously outlined for an effective drug treatment. Continuing research into this substance with longer follow-up periods is therefore justified, taking account of the following points:

(1) An antiandrogen (e.g. CPA) should be given concurrently, at least in the first month. Any abrupt withdrawal must be avoided because of a possible rebound effect[17,21].

(2) Checking the efficacy is complex. Blood testosterone levels and the incidence of reoffending are taken as 'objective variables'. However, it is the subjects' own assessments that primarily enable the effect on fantasies and behavior to be evaluated. It would make sense to use uniform, standardized questionnaires to aid comparability between studies.

(3) So far studies have mainly dealt with pedophilia subjects (80% of the total of 41 participants). We are also interested in whether there is any therapeutic effect in less common forms of paraphilia (e.g. sadomasochism).

(4) On the question of efficacy, there is no alternative to controlled trials.

REFERENCES

1. Walther S. Umgang mit Sexualstraftäter: Amerika, Quo vadis? Vergewisserung über aktuelle Grundfragen an das (deutsche) Strafrecht. *Monatsschr Kriminol Strafrechtsreform* 1997;80:199–221
2. Dilling H, Mombour W, Schmidt MH, eds. *Internationale Klassifikation psychischer Störungen*. ICD 10, Kapitel V (F), klinisch-diagnostische Leitlinien, Weltgesundheitsorganisation. Bern, Göttingen, Toronto: Huber, 1991
3. Saß J, Wittchen H-U, Zaudig M. *Diagnostisches und statistisches Manual psychischer Störungen DSM-IV (dt. Bearb.)*. Göttingen: Hogrefe, 1996
4. Statistisches Bundesamt. Strafverfolgung. Rechtspflege, Fachserie 10, Reihe 3, 1996
5. Statistisches Bundesamt. Strafvollzug – Demographische und kriminologische Merkmale von Strafgefangenen am 31.03.1997. Rechtspflege, Fachserie 10, Reihe 4.1, 1997
6. Wille R, Beier KM. Nachuntersuchungen von kastrierten Sexualstraftätern. *Sexuologie* 1997;4:1–26
7. Hall GCN. Sexual offenders recidivism revisited: a meta-analysis of recent treatment studies. *J Consult Clin Psychol* 1995;63:902–8
8. Laschet U, Laschet L. Psychopharmacotherapy of sex offenders with cyproterone acetate. *Pharmakopsychiatrie Neuropsychopharmakol* 1971;4:99–104
9. Ahrens R. Androcur (Cyproteronacetat) bei Sexualdelinquenz – Nachuntersuchung von untergebrachten psychiatrischen Patienten. *Schweiz Arch Neurol Psychiatrie* 1991;142:171–88
10. Menghini P, Ernst K. Die Antiandrogenbehandlung im rückblickenden Urteil von 19 Sexualstraftätern. *Nervenarzt* 1991;62:303–7
11. Cooper AJ, Cernovsky ZZ. The effects of cyproterone acetate on sleeping and waking penile erections in pedophiles: possible implications for treatment. *Can J Psychiatr* 1992;37:33–9
12. Gijs L, Gooren L. Hormonal and psychopharmacological interventions in the treatment of paraphilias: an update. *J Sex Res* 1996;33:273–90
13. Bradford JMW, Greenberg DM. Pharmacological treatment of deviant sexual behaviour. *Annu Rev Sex Res* 1996;7:283–305
14. Heller CG, Laidlaw MW, Harvey HT, Nelson DL. The effects of the progestational compounds of the reproductive processes of the human male. *Ann NY Acad Sci* 1958;71:649–55
15. Meyer WJ, Collier C, Emory E. Depo provera treatment for sex offending behaviour. An evaluation of outcome. *Bull Am Acad Psychiatr Law* 1992;20:249–59
16. Allolio B, Keffel D, Deuss U, Winkelmann W. Behandlung sexueller Verhaltensstörungen mit LH-RH-Superagonisten. *Dtsch Med Wochenschr* 1985;110:1952
17. Rousseau L, Couture M, Dupont A, Labrie F, Couture N. Effect of combined androgen blockade with LHRH agonist and flutamide in one severe case of male exhibitionism. *Can J Psychiatr* 1990;35:338–41
18. Dickey R. The management of a case of treatment-resistant paraphilia with a longacting LHRH agonist. *Can J Psychiatr* 1992;37:567–9
19. Marcus AO, Fernandez MP, De Keyser L. Use of gonadotropin releasing hormone analog in treatment of exhibitionism. *Clin Res* 1993;41:107A

20. Cooper AJ, Cernovsky ZZ. Comparison of cyproterone acetate (CPA) and leuprolide acetate (LHRH agonist) in a chronic pedophile: a clinical case study. *Biol Psychiatr* 1994;36:269–71
21. Thibaut F, Cordier B, Kuhn JM. Effect of a long-lasting gonadotropin hormone-releasing hormone agonist in six cases of severe male paraphilia. *Acta Psychiatr Scand* 1993;87:445–50
22. Thibaut F, Cordier B, Kuhn JM. Gonadotropin hormone-releasing hormone agonist in cases of severe male paraphilia: a lifetime treatment? *Psychoneuroendocrinology* 1996;21:409–11
23. Rösler A, Witztum E. Treatment of men with paraphilia with a long-acting analogue of gonadotropin-releasing hormone. *N Engl J Med* 1998;12:416–22

7
Pathogenesis and medical management of uterine fibroids

I. A. Brosens and B. Lunenfeld

INTRODUCTION

Uterine fibroids represent the most common tumor in women. The development of fibroids after the menarche, the enlargement and growth during reproductive life and the regression after menopause suggest that the growth depends on the ovarian steroids, estrogens and progesterone. Although surgery has been the treatment of choice for conservative and permanent treatment, there are more and more circumstances in which medical treatment would be more than welcome. For this reason, a symposium was organized to evaluate the state of knowledge regarding the pathogenesis and the possibilities of medical management.

HISTOGENESIS AND GROWTH

The theory of Meyer[1] that the cells of uterine leiomyoma originate from myoblasts of the musculature has been rather generally accepted. However, the myoblasts which are to become the progenitors of leiomyoma have not been identified. Dr Shingo Fujii and collaborators [1] have analyzed leiomyomatosis peritonealis disseminata (LPD), experimental LPD, smooth muscle cell development in the human fetal uterus and the proliferative mechanisms of myometrial smooth muscle cell proliferation during the reproductive period. From there, they have identified two different candidates as potential progenitors of leiomyomas: the undifferentiated mesenchymal cell and the myometrial smooth muscle cell. Their recent investigations with advanced molecular techniques, however, suggest that the myometrial smooth muscle cell itself is a likely candidate to be the progenitor of uterine leiomyomas. A leiomyoma may arise from a single parent cell derived from smooth muscle elements of the myometrium, involving somatic mutations and the complex interactions of reproductive steroids and local growth factors and cytokines during the repetition of the menstrual cycle.

Dr T. Maruo and collaborators [2] examined how sex steroids influence the proliferation of leiomyoma cells. As epidermal growth factor (EGF) has been shown to mediate estrogen action, they investigated the effects of sex steroids on the expression of EGF and EGF-receptor (EGF-R) in leiomyoma cells. In cultures of leiomyoma cells, they could show that progesterone upregulates the expression of proliferating cell nuclear antigen (PCNA) and EGF in leiomyoma cells, whereas estradiol upregulates the expression of PCNA and EGF-R. It is, therefore, conceivable that estradiol and progesterone act in combination to stimulate the proliferative potential of leiomyoma cells through the induction of EGF and EGF-R expression.

The authors also found that Bcl-2 protein, an apoptosis-inhibiting gene product, was abundantly present in leiomyoma in comparison with normal myometrium and that Bcl-2 protein expression in leiomyoma cells was upregulated by progesterone, but down-regulated by estradiol. It seems, therefore, likely that progesterone may also participate in leiomyoma growth through the induction of Bcl-2 protein in leiomyoma cells. The abundant expression of Bcl-2 protein in leiomyoma may be one of the molecular bases for the enhanced growth of leiomyoma in comparison to that of normal myometrium.

MOLECULAR BIOLOGY

The role played by estrogen and progestin receptors in mediating the effects of ovarian sex steroids in target organs is now well established. More elusive is a molecular definition of the factors that determine tissue-specific responses to systematic estradiol and progesterone, and how within the uterus, for example, it is possible to achieve such spatial and temporal diversity to hormonal stimulation. In the endometrium, the phenotypical responsiveness is minimal in the basal layer and gradually increases towards the endometrial surface. The zonal differentiation of the response to ovarian hormones also differentiates the human myometrium into the subendometrial layer, or junctional zone, and the outer myometrial layer. The spatial and temporal expression of uterine target genes in response to the estrogen and progesterone of uterine target genes cannot be explained merely on the basis of differential expression of their cognate receptors. Growing evidence suggests that these orchestrated responses require interaction between steroid hormone receptors and cell surface signalling pathways activated by locally produced factors. Downstream signalling intermediates of growth factors and cytokine molecules can determine the cellular response to steroid hormones.

Dr Jan Brosens [3] proposed different levels of cross-talk between cell surface signal transduction pathways and nuclear receptors. First, all receptors are phosphoproteins and targeted phosphorylation by cellular kinases has been shown to modulate receptor function and even results in transactivation of the receptor in the absence of ligand. Second, nuclear receptors can directly interact with other transcription factors, thus resulting in repression or enhancement of progesterone receptor (PR) transactivation potential. Third, most coactivators and corepressors are promiscuous proteins which can bind to a plethora of nuclear receptors and other transcription factors. Hence, the transactivation or transrepression potential of a steroid receptor can be limited through competition with other transcription factors for a finite pool of cofactors. Fourth, evidence is emerging to indicate that liganded steroid receptors can activate components of cytoplasmic signalling and thereby sensitize cells to the actions of extracellular signalling molecules. Finally, tissue recombination studies, using wild-type and steroid receptor knock-out mice, have yielded important insights into the paracrine role of PR and ERα in uterine tissues. Admittedly, the mechanisms of cross-talk between nuclear receptors and other transcriptional factors have been studied almost exclusively in model cell lines and, hence, the relevance of many of these interactions in uterine physiology and pathophysiology remains largely to be determined.

Dr Steven Smith [4] has discussed new insights into the factors involved in the angiogenesis in fibroids and endometrium. Agents that are involved in the proliferation of vascular smooth muscle, including the insulin-like growth factor (IGF) family of genes, at least with respect to IGF-II, but not IGF-I, are elevated in fibroids. Similarly, agents which promote angiogenesis, such as vascular endothelial growth factor, are also elevated in fibroids, raising the possibility that the angiogenesis associated with the endometrium overlying submucosal fibroids and in the surrounding myometrium may arise because of overexpression of angiogenic growth factors. The observation, that gonadotropin releasing hormone (GnRH) agonists may exert direct effects on myometrial proliferation via the transforming growth factor family of growth factors, taken in conjunction with the above information, raises the possibility that regulation of growth factor expression and/or receptors may in the future provide new means of regulating fibroid growth. Advances in our understanding of the basic science of angiogenesis could potentially lead to mechanisms of intervention to prevent disease progression.

CYTOGENETICS

Dr Paola Dal Cin [5] has investigated for many years the cytogenetics of benign solid tumors and described our present knowledge of the cytogenetics of the uterine leiomyoma. About 40% are karyotypically abnormal. At least five major cytogenetically abnormal subgroups have been identified: involvement of 12q15 and 6p21, interstitial deletions of chromosome regions 7q and 3q and trisomy 12. However, other aberrations can also be observed such as r(1) and involvement of 10q, t(1;2). This variety of cytogenetic subgroups indicates involvement of different genes. Two genes have already been identified, and are directly involved, at least in those leiomyomas characterized by rearrangements of 12q15 and 6p21. These two genes, HMGI-C and HMGI-(Y), respectively, belong to the high-mobility group of proteins which are accessory transcription factors, and are also involved in other benign mesenchymal tumors carrying the same cytogenetic aberrations. A clue to the nature of the genes, probably tumor suppressor ones, involved in the interstitial deletion of chromosomes 7 and 3, is not yet available.

Both genes HMGI-C and HMGI-(Y) are predominantly expressed during embryonic development and are thought to be involved in cell differentiation and proliferation processes. Therefore, it was suggested that HMGI-C and HMGI-(Y) might be involved in the neoplastic transformation of uterine leiomyomas. To find out whether HMGI gene expression is induced in uterine leiomyomas, Dr Ulrike Fuhrmann [6] has analyzed primary tumor tissues in comparison to the corresponding normal myometrium by Western blot analysis. Sixteen out of 33 analyzed uterine leiomyomas expressed high levels of HMGI-C or HMGI-(Y), while both proteins were not detected in normal uterine myometrium. The results of Western blot analysis could be confirmed by Northern blot analysis and immunohistochemistry. Three of the analyzed uterine leiomyomas expressed HMGI-C proteins and mRNAs with abnormal molecular weight, indicating that they were made from chimeric genes generated by chromosomal rearrangements. All other HMGI-positive tumors expressed HMGI gene products of the predicted molecular weight. Based on these data, the author suggested that the induction of the expression of functionally active HMGI proteins, rather than the expression of chimeric HMGI proteins, is crucial for the pathogenesis of uterine leiomyomas.

BASIC CLINICAL FEATURES

Dr A. Schindler [7] has reviewed the recent epidemiological data. A recent prospective study confirmed an inverse relationship with parity and age at first birth and a positive relationship with years since last birth and history of infertility. The use of sonography in epidemiological studies has shown a more than quadruplication of the incidence of fibroids with age. Sonographic studies in the Hiroshima atomic bomb survivors showed a dose–response relationship. Family studies found a significant increase in first-degree relatives within families where there were two or more family members with fibroids. Cigarette smoking seems to reduce the risk of fibroids. The effect of hormonal contraception remains controversial, except that there might be a risk reduction when hormonal contraceptives are taken for more than 10 years and with the use of high-dose medroxyprogesterone acetate.

Progress in sonography is likely to benefit greatly the medical management of uterine fibroids. Dr Asim Kurjak and Dr Sanya Kupesic [8] studied extensively the uterine blood flow and uterine leiomyoma blood supply. Increased blood flow velocity and decreased resistance index and pulsatility index in both uterine arteries occurred in patients with uterine leiomyomas. In the main arteries supplying identifiable leiomyomas, the diastolic flow was always present and was increased in comparison with uterine artery blood flow. The difference in uterine artery blood flow between patients with vascularized leiomyomas and healthy volunteers is significant and may be used for prediction of the growth rate of these tumors. It is expected that integrated software for calculating the total extent of vascularity in a three-dimensional perspective will allow determination of the total tumor perfusion.

From clinical experience, we know that uterine fibroids are not a homogeneous group and that there is considerable variation of pattern of growth and response to GnRH agonist treatment from case to case and from tumor to tumor. Dr Ivo Brosens and collaborators [9] further analyzed the correlation between size and cytogenetic abnormalities. Recent data suggest that specific chromosomal abnormalities within individual fibroids may alter sex steroid hormone dependency and modify the growth of the tumor as well as the response to GnRH agonist treatment. Fibroids originating from the subendometrial myometrium or junctional zone, or submucous fibroids, also differ in their pathophysiology from fibroids of the outer myometrium. They express higher levels of sex steroid hormone receptors, have an identifiable artery at sonography more frequently and show significantly less cytogenetic abnormalities. Clinical data also suggest that the spontaneous growth rate of submucous fibroids is lower, but the response to GnRH agonists is higher than that of fibroids in the outer myometrium.

HORMONAL THERAPY
Pretreatment in fibroid surgery

GnRH analogue therapy is now well established as pretreatment in hysteroscopic fibroid surgery. Submucosal fibroids are classified using hysterosalpingography into three categories:

(1) Submucosal fibroids with their greatest diameter inside the uterine cavity (type I);

(2) Submucosal fibroids with their largest portion in the uterine wall (type II);

(3) Multiple submucosal fibroids (type III).

The surgical technique is adapted according to the type. A large type II fibroid can be treated in two surgical steps. The first step is resection of the intracavitary portion and fiber laser coagulation of the intramural portion, and the second step is performed after the continuing use of GnRH analogue results in the intracavitary protrusion of the intramural part. The mechanism of expulsion during GnRH analogue therapy is remarkable and apparently leaves no scar in the wall. It is obvious that, after surgery of type III fibroids, recurrences are frequent and that GnRH analogues may result in masking small submucosal fibroids.

In a series of 244 women, Nisolle and collaborators [10] found an average shrinkage of 38% after 8 weeks of treatment with an injectable GnRH agonist. However, the shrinkage varied from 4 to 95%, and in 10% no shrinkage was seen. In 1%, a malignant stromal tumor was present, which underlines the need for histological diagnosis. It is assumed that lack of shrinkage can suggest malignancy, but, on the other hand, shrinkage during GnRH analogue treatment has been described in uterine sarcomas.

The advantages of the pre-operative use of GnRH analogues are:

(1) Reduction of size;

(2) Decreased risk of fluid overload during hysteroscopic surgery;

(3) Normalization of hemoglobin concentration;

(4) Evaluation of the response of the tumor.

Long-term GnRH analogue treatment

Early observations by Dr Rodolphe Maheux [11] showed that uterine fibroids regressed during GnRH analogue treatment, even if estrogen levels were not completely suppressed. To conserve some estrogen level, add-back therapy has been more practical than titration of the dosage of GnRH analogue. Estrogen/progestin is usually added after the first 3 months of GnRH analogue therapy. A continuous regimen is preferred over a cyclic one, as it is associated with less bleeding and hot flushes. GnRH analogues with add-back can effectively control the symptomatology of fibroids with minimal side-effects. However, the regimen has never been as popular for fibroids as for endometriosis, probably because other solutions, more practical or offering a permanent solution, are now available. Recurrence is the rule when treatment is stopped. Oral contraceptives significantly reduce menstruation and dysmenorrhea and now can be used for non-smokers up to the time of menopause. Endoscopic surgery now also offers a range of alternative procedures to conventional hysterectomy from which to choose according to the clinical condition: hysteroscopic myomectomy with or without endometrial ablation, laparoscopic myomectomy and supracervical hysterectomy. GnRH analogues with add-back therapy should therefore be seen as a second-line therapy in patients with fibroids.

GnRH antagonists

The use of GnRH agonists in the preoperative treatment of fibroids is logical as it may shorten the duration of treatment necessary for obtaining shrinkage of the tumor. In a phase-II study using a depot preparation of the third-generation gonadotropin releasing hormone antagonist cetrorelix (SB-75) involving 20 patients, Felberbaum and colleagues showed that the treatment of fibroids is feasible and effective [13]. A maximal reduction was achieved within 14 days of treatment, which is faster than when using an agonist preparation. The ovarian function can be restored in shorter times, compared to treatment with a GnRH agonist depot. However, the effectiveness was only found in a subgroup of patients, as 37% of the patients showed a poor response regarding the reduction of the uterine volume and 15% dropped out due to side-effects. Further pharmacological improvements are necessary to reduce the present disadvantages.

Antiestrogens and antiprogestogens

Dr Jacques Donnez [12] examined whether antiestrogens may be the key therapy during the next millennium. Tamoxifen is featured as an antiestrogen, but its agonistic estrogen action should not be ignored. In addition to the well-known risks of endometrial hyperplasia, endometrial polyps and endometrial cancer developing in women receiving tamoxifen treatment, there have now been reports of fibroids appearing or worsening during tamoxifen therapy. An antiestrogen without any agonist action, under the code name of ICI 182,780, is now available for investigation. The compound is well tolerated in short-term use and appears to have a potent antiestrogenic effect on the endometrium. A multicenter European phase II study is under way.

Given the concept of progesterone action upon fibroids mentioned above, the use of an antiprogesterone in the treatment of fibroids merits further study according to Dr Etienne Baulieu [14], inventor of RU486. The product has been shown by the group of Dr S. S. C. Yen[2] to cause a regression of myoma volume at least as important as that obtained with GnRH agonists, but with maintenance of estrogen levels. This is obtained with a dose of 25 mg/day, which does not significantly alter the pituitary–adrenal system. Well-monitored trials, however, are required before long-term use can be recommended.

REFERENCES

1. Meyer R. *Die pathologische Anatomie der Gebarmutter, Handbuch der speziellen pathologischen Anatomie und Histologie*. Berlin: Springer Verlag, 1930;VII/I:213–49
2. Murphy AA, Kettel LM, Morales AJ, *et al*. Regression of uterine leiomyomata in response to the antiprogesterone RU486. *J Clin Endocrinol Metab* 1993;76:513–17

BIBLIOGRAPHY

Abstracts of relevant papers presented at the 5th International Symposium on GnRH Analogues in Cancer and Human Reproduction

1. Mesenchymal cell differentiation. S. Fujii, I. Konishi, A. Horiuchi, A. Orii, T. Nikaido, Japan
2. Sex steroidal regulation of leiomyoma growth and apoptosis: its relevance to the treatment with GnRH agonists. T. Maruo, H. Matsuo, T. Samoto, Y. Shimomura, O. Kurachi, S. Mochizuki, Japan
3. Sex steroid hormone action. J. Brosens, I. Mak, J. White, UK
4. Growth factors. S.K. Smith, UK
5. Cytogenetics. P. Dal Cin, Belgium
6. Expression of high mobility group I proteins in uterine leiomyomas. U. Fuhrmann, A. Waßerfall, M. Klotzbucher, Germany
7. Epidemiology of uterine fibroids. A.E. Schindler, Germany
8. 3D and color Doppler imaging of uterine fibroids. A. Kurjak, S. Kupesic, Croatia
9. Clinico-pathological features of uterine leiomyomas. I. Brosens, P. Dal Cin, J. Deprest, H. Van den Berghe, Belgium
10. GnRH-agonist as pretreatment in fibroid surgery. M. Nisolle, S. Gillerot, M. Berlière, F. Casanas-Roux, J. Donnez, Belgium
11. GnRH agonist and add-back therapy. R. Maheux, Canada
12. Progestogens and antiestrogens. J. Donnez, Belgium
13. Medical management of uterine fibroids: GnRH antagonists. R.E. Felberbaum, Germany
14. A role for the antiprogestin mifepristone (RU 486) in the treatment of uterine leiomyoma. E.-E. Baulieu, France

8
GnRH analogues in the management of endometriosis:
K.W. Schweppe

Although gonadotropin releasing hormone analogues (GnRHa) were introduced as a new approach for the treatment of endometriosis 17 years ago[1], there is no consensus about the exact role of these substances in the management of this disease. Choosing an optimal treatment for a woman with endometriosis is difficult, because it requires first, an understanding of the cause and development of the disease; second, an understanding of the therapeutic options; and finally, the fact that individual expectations of the patients – pain or pregnancy – have to be taken into account.

UNDERSTANDING ENDOMETRIOSIS

Tremendous research has been done on endometriosis over the past seven decades, but the etiology is still unclear and the pathophysiology is only partly understood. Endometriosis is characterized by a large variety of symptoms, which can also occur in patients without endometriosis; sometimes, patients with endometriosis do not have symptoms at all. Endometriotic implants have a wide spectrum of macroscopic and microscopic appearances and they differ in their biochemical activities. The type of growth has a wide spectrum too – whether it is peritoneal disease, ovarian involvement or deep infiltrating endometriosis in the cul-de-sac or the rectovaginal septum. Donnez and co-workers[2] have proposed that these different types of organ involvement express three different entities of the disease, each needing different treatment strategies.

UNDERSTANDING THERAPEUTIC OPTIONS

Surgical and medical therapy or a combination of both are the treatment options today. Many non-comparative studies involving radical, classical conservative treatment via laparotomy and endoscopic surgery with only short follow-up have been poorly validated, because large randomized studies with adequate follow-up are lacking. Up to now the best data have come from the Canadian multicenter study published by Marcoux and co-workers[3], demonstrating a significant benefit for endoscopic surgery. For deep infiltrating endometriosis and ovarian endometriomata this seems to be the only option. Radical surgery is for most women not an option, unless it is absolutely necessary. Resection or vaporization of implants, cysts or deep infiltrating nodules or even removal of the involved organ are effective in controlling the disease and its symptoms, but they do not provide a cure, and, for the majority of patients, the disease and its symptoms recur.

GnRHa, danazol, oral contraceptives and progestins reduce pelvic pain and resolve endometrial implants in a large number of women whilst being administered, but after cessation of medication there is – depending on the stage of the disease – a high recurrence rate of up to 70% within 5 years. Repeated medication and/or a combination of medical and endoscopic surgery has therefore to be taken into account. For these reasons, the efficacy of a substance with respect to regression of implants and reduction of symptoms is important, but also the spectrum and the degree of side-effects must be judged, when the drug must be administered over a long period or repeatedly. Ranking existing medical treatments in order of side-effects – from the least disliked to the most disliked substance – GnRHa with add-back medication are the first choice, progestins are middle and danazol is the last ranking.

UNDERSTANDING PATIENTS' EXPECTATIONS

In the patient with pelvic pain, dysmenorrhea, dyspareunia and other uncharacteristic lower abdominal or back pain caused by endometriosis, the primary goal is a correct diagnosis, as stated by the Endometriosis Association. In general, it takes more than 5 years from the onset of symptoms to the correct diagnosis. This has to be improved, especially when we see the data from Schindler [55] demonstrating that early stages of endometriosis show higher metabolic, immunological and mitotic activity with prostaglandin and cytokine expression than do later stages. Therefore, early disease reacts better to hormonal deprivation (e.g. with GnRHa) than do more advanced stages. The absolute recurrence rate is lower and the recurrence-free interval is longer for early stages of active endometriosis in comparison with advanced stages in which therapeutic approaches are used. The treatment goal in these patients is pain relief with regression of endometriosis.

GnRHa are more effective than progestins, as confirmed by a prospective randomized study of Schindler and colleagues [58]. GnRHa with add-back medication are safe, effective and well tolerated, as confirmed by Aono and associates [49] who used conjugated estrogen and medroxyprogesterone acetate in the add-back group and leuprorelin acetate alone in the control group. The add-back therapy significantly prevented bone mineral density reduction, and the Kupperman indices were significantly lower.

Different GnRHa are similarly effective in reducing pelvic symptoms associated with endometriosis, as confirmed by Shaw and co-workers [51] for leuprorelin and triptorelin. In addition, different GnRHa were similarly effective in regression of implants and 50% of patients still had residual foci containing glands and stroma at the end of a 6-month treatment period, which was shown morphologically by Ruwe and colleagues [54] for leuprorelin and buserelin.

GnRHa medication can be repeated if the patient has recurrent disease. Although Ayabe and co-workers [50] reported a recurrence rate of 17.8% only 1 year after treatment with buserelin 900 μg daily, we know from larger studies[4] that the recurrence rates are stage related and as high as 70% after 3 years for progressed disease. Therefore, the information from Uemura and associates [56] is very important. The demineralization was less in the second course of GnRHa administration than in the first course. They concluded that 'selection of patients, sufficient interval and optimal dosage of GnRH agonist diminish the risk of bone loss in patients treated with GnRH agonists repeatedly'. We can add that the use of add-back medication will further diminish the risk and makes repeated, intermittent or even continuous treatment with GnRHa possible.

Guidelines for clinical practice in the management of patients with endometriosis-related pain is given in Figure 1. In minimal disease diagnostic laparoscopy should be expanded to endoscopic surgery using vaporization, high frequency or endothermic coagulation to destroy the visible implants. In case of active disease residual microscopic implants will probably be responsible for recurrences and should then be treated with medication. In progressed stages it is often difficult to restore the reproductive organs completely, therefore medical treatment followed by sufficient endoscopic surgery may be the best, as demonstrated for ovarian cysts by Donnez and associates[5].

For the patient with infertility, the management of infertility associated with the chronic, recurrent disease of endometriosis remains controversial. In severe and extensive cases organ damage and adhesions represent mechanical causes of infertility; however, mild and minimal disease can be associated with functional infertility or can be regarded as a chance finding. GnRHa used alone or in

```
                    ┌─────────────────────┐
                    │ Diagnostic pelviscopy│
                    └──────────┬──────────┘
              ┌────────────────┴────────────────┐
              ▼                                 ▼
     ┌─────────────────┐              ┌─────────────────┐
     │ Pelviscopic surgery│           │  Active disease │
     └────────┬────────┘              └────────┬────────┘
              ▼                                 ▼
 ┌─────────────────────────┐        ┌─────────────────────────┐
 │ Recurrence of symptoms  │        │    Medical treatment    │
 │ Symptomatic medical     │        │    GnRHa 3–6 months     │
 │ treatment               │        │ Danazol or high-dose    │
 │                         │        │ progestins              │
 └───────────┬─────────────┘        └────────────┬────────────┘
             ▼                                   ▼
 ┌─────────────────────────┐        ┌─────────────────────────┐
 │ Analgesics              │        │    Repeat pelviscopy    │
 │ Oral contraceptives     │───────▶│ Suspected recurrence of │
 │ Progestins              │        │ endometriosis           │
 │                         │        │ Symptomatic therapy     │
 │                         │        │ insufficient            │
 └─────────────────────────┘        └─────────────────────────┘
```

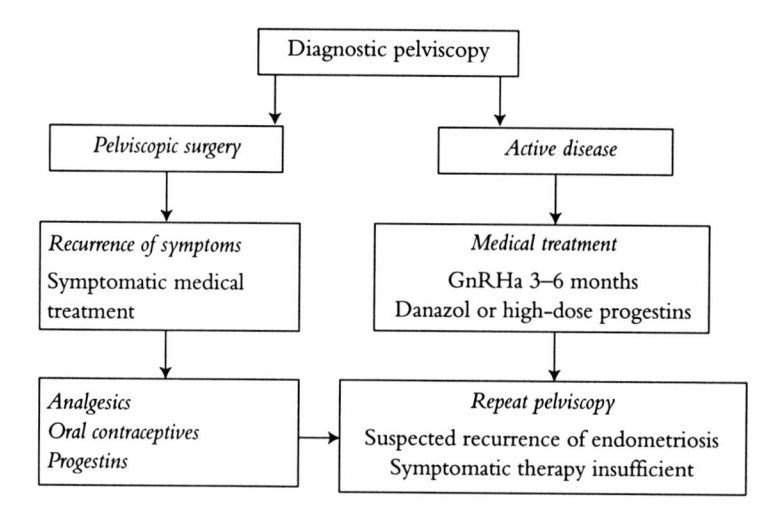

Figure 1 Management of patients with endometriosis and pain and the place of GnRHa in the therapeutic strategy

combination with endoscopic surgery not only gives symptomatic pain relief and reduction of size and extent of the endometriotic implants, but also results in pregnancies in previously infertile patients. Down-regulation with GnRHa prior to stimulation in *in vitro* fertilization (IVF) protocols has resulted in the prevention of premature luteinizing hormone (LH) surges, more oocytes and an improvement of pregnancy rates compared with non-GnRHa protocols. Radwanska from Chicago presented a study [57] evaluating the effects of GnRHa in intrauterine insemination (IUI) or IVF cycles in 230 women with endometriosis. Among patients undergoing IVF, increasing the duration of leuprorelin suppression led to increased cycle fecundity in up to 38% with suppression longer than 3 months. A similar increase up to 21% was seen in patients undergoing IUI cycles.

For the practical management of an infertile patient with endometriosis the guidelines are illustrated in Figure 2. Primarily minimal disease – especially if the macroscopic and microscopic appearances correspond to inactive lesions – should not be considered as a factor reducing fecundity. If other infertility factors are excluded or corrected and stimulation of ovarian function does not result in a pregnancy after six cycles, endometriosis can be accepted as a cause of infertility and the disease should be treated medically. After cessation of medication ovarian stimulation is indicated again for 6–9 cycles. If no pregnancy occurs, repeat pelviscopy can be performed because of suspected recurrent endometriosis. In that case endoscopic excision or vaporization of the foci is recommended, because the endometriotic implant has not responded to medical treatment sufficiently. In severe stages

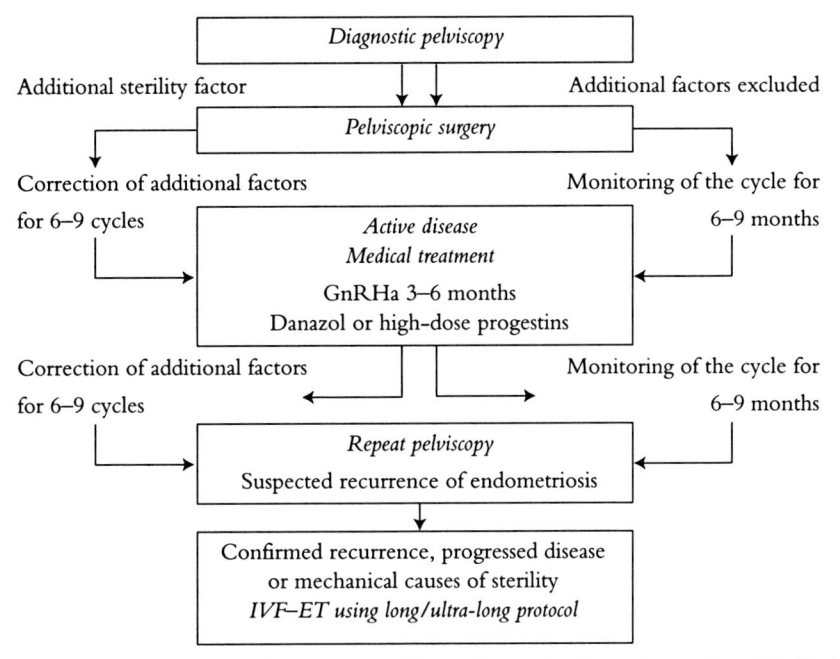

```
                    ┌─────────────────────────┐
                    │  Diagnostic pelviscopy  │
                    └─────────────────────────┘
  Additional sterility factor  │   │  Additional factors excluded
              ┌────────────────┘   └────────────────┐
              ▼                                      ▼
         ┌─────────────────────────────┐
         │     Pelviscopic surgery     │
         └─────────────────────────────┘
 Correction of additional factors        Monitoring of the cycle for
        for 6–9 cycles                           6–9 months
              │    ┌──────────────────────┐    │
              └───▶│    Active disease    │◀───┘
                   │   Medical treatment  │
                   │   GnRHa 3–6 months   │
                   │ Danazol or high-dose │
                   │      progestins      │
                   └──────────────────────┘
 Correction of additional factors        Monitoring of the cycle for
        for 6–9 cycles                           6–9 months
              │    ┌──────────────────────┐    │
              └───▶│   Repeat pelviscopy  │◀───┘
                   │ Suspected recurrence │
                   │   of endometriosis   │
                   └──────────────────────┘
                              │
                              ▼
              ┌──────────────────────────────────┐
              │ Confirmed recurrence, progressed │
              │ disease or mechanical causes of  │
              │             sterility            │
              │ IVF–ET using long/ultra-long     │
              │            protocol              │
              └──────────────────────────────────┘
```

Figure 2 Management of patients with endometriosis and associated infertility and the place of GnRHa in the therapeutic strategy

endoscopic surgery must remove the cysts and implants and restore the reproductive organs. If surgery is incomplete, post-surgical treatment is recommended. If surgery and medical treatment have failed, assisted reproduction using GnRHa with the long or ultra-long protocol will give the best chance of achieving a pregnancy.

These facts characterize the state of our knowledge about GnRHa and endometriosis based on the results of the 5th International Symposium on GnRH Analogues today. Further studies are necessary to reach understanding of the disease with respect to active and inactive lesions and with respect to the differences of peritoneal involvement, ovarian cysts and deep infiltrating endometriosis. Further prospective randomized trials are also necessary to evaluate the therapeutic options with respect to medical therapy prior to or after surgery and with respect to endometriosis and infertility.

REFERENCES

1. Meldrun DR, Chang RJ, Lu J, *et al*. Medical oophorectomy using a long-acting GnRH agonist: a possible new approach to the treatment of endometriosis. *J Clin Endocrinol Metab* 1982;54:1081–3

2. Donnez J, Nissole M, Smoes P, Gillet N, Beguin S, Casanas-Roux F. Peritoneal endometriosis and 'endometriotic' nodules of the rectovaginal septum are two different entities. *Fertil Steril* 1996;66:362–8
3. Marcoux S, Maheux R, Berube S. Laparoscopic surgery in infertile women with minimal or mild endometriosis. Canadian Collaborative Group on Endometriosis. *N Engl J Med* 1997;337:217–22
4. Waller KG, Shaw RW. Gonodotropin-releasing hormone analogue for the treatment of endometriosis: long term follow up. *Fertil Steril* 1993;59:511–15
5. Donnez J, Nisolle M, Gillerot S, Anaf V, Clerckx-Braun F, Casanas-Roux F. Ovarian endometrial cysts: the role of gonadotropin-releasing hormone agonist and/or drainage. *Fertil Steril* 1994;62:63–6

BIBLIOGRAPHY

Abstracts of relevant papers presented at the 5th International Symposium on GnRH Analogues in Cancer and Human Reproduction

49. The efficacy of add-back therapy with every other day administration of both CEE and MPA in patients with endometriosis. T. Aono, N. Yoneda, T. Yasui, K. Azuma, M. Irahara, Japan
50. Recurrence rate at one year after the treatment of endometriosis by nasal administration of buserelin acetate: multicentral study in Japan. T. Ayabe, H. Mori, Y. Taketani, T. Uemura, A. Miyake, T. Tango, Japan
51. Triptorelin vs. leuprorelin for treatment of pelvic pain associated with endometriosis: a randomised study. R.W. Shaw, P. Dewart, E. Thomas, *et al.*, UK
54. Endometriosis: clinical, histological and morphometrical results before and after GnRH-agonist therapy. M. Ruwe, K. Donhuijsen, P.A. Regidor, L.D. Leder, A.E. Schindler, Germany
55. Early treatment of endometriosis with GnRH-agonists: impact on symptoms, reproduction and quality of life. A.E. Schindler, Germany
56. Effects of retreatment with GnRH agonists on bone mineral density in patients with endometriosis. T. Uemura, H. Yoshikata, M. Ishikawa, Y. Kondoh, N. Hirahara, H. Minaguchi, Japan
57. The effect of GnRH agonist suppression on the outcome of infertility treatment in women with endometriosis. E. Radwanska, USA
58. Comparison of leuprorelin vs. lynestrenol in patients with endometriosis. A.E. Schindler, P.A. Regidor, G. Lübben, E. Kienle, P. Förtig, Germany

9
GnRH analogues in ovarian, breast and endometrial cancers

S. Westphalen and G. Emons

INTRODUCTION

The application of gonadotropin releasing hormone (GnRH) analogues (GnRHa) in the therapy of cancers of the ovary, the breast and the endometrium is based on four potential pharmacological mechanisms of these peptides:

(1) GnRHa-induced selective medical hypophysectomy (suppression of gonadotropin secretion), which has been suggested to be of value in the therapy of ovarian cancer;

(2) GnRHa-induced medical ovariectomy (suppression of ovarian secretion of estrogens and progestins), which has become an established therapy of disseminated, estrogen-dependent breast cancer in pre- and perimenopausal women;

(3) GnRH receptor-mediated direct anti-tumor effects in breast, ovarian and endometrial cancer cells;

(4) Use of GnRHa as carriers for cytotoxic radicals possibly allowing targeted chemotherapy of breast, ovarian and endometrial cancers expressing receptors for GnRH.

Since the 4th International Symposium on GnRH Analogues in Cancer and Human Reproduction in Geneva in February 1996[1], many new important preclinical and clinical data have been published on the use of GnRHa in ovarian, breast and endometrial cancers. These results and the latest data presented at the 5th International Symposium on GnRH Analogues in Cancer and Human Reproduction in Geneva in February 1999 will be reviewed here.

RESULTS OF RECENT PRECLINICAL RESEARCH

Expression of GnRH receptors and GnRH in ovarian, breast and endometrial cancers

The expression of GnRH and its receptor as well as direct antiproliferative effects of GnRHa have been demonstrated in human ovarian, breast and endometrial cancers[2].

In recent years convincing evidence has been accumulated that GnRH directly affects cancers of various extra-pituitary tissues such as the ovary, breast, endometrium and prostate. It is likely that a GnRH-based autocrine system is present in a number of human malignant tumors. Interfering with growth factors and growth factor receptors, this GnRH system might be involved in negative autocrine regulation of proliferation of these tumor cells (for review see Chapter 1) [23, 65][2-7].

GnRH immunoreactivity was detected in biopsy samples of human breast cancer[8] as well as in breast cancer cell lines[9]. Subsequently the expression of GnRH messenger RNA was demonstrated in human breast cancer cell lines[10].

Significant amounts of GnRH immunoreactivity were described in ovarian cancer biopsies and in the ovarian cancer cell line SKOV-3[11] as well as in extracts of the human ovarian cancer cell lines EFO-21 and EFO-27[12]. This GnRH immunoreactivity is biologically active[11,12]. In addition, GnRH mRNA has been detected in these specimens[11,12].

Comparable data on GnRH immunoreactivity, bioactivity and mRNA have been collected in the human endometrial cancer cell lines HEC-1A and Ishikawa and in endometrial cancer samples[13-15].

Corresponding to these findings, GnRH receptors have been shown to be expressed in about 80% of human ovarian and endometrial carcinomas and in about 50% of breast cancers [62][14,16-20]. In addition to these findings in human breast cancers [62][16,17,20], GnRH receptors have been demonstrated in normal breast tissue [62][20] and in human breast cancer cell lines[21-24].

Human ovarian and endometrial cancer cell lines as well as biopsy samples express two different types of GnRH receptors, one of high affinity and low capacity and one of low affinity and high capacity in about 80% of the cases[2,4,12,13,18,19,25-27].

Major findings about the biological function and the signalling pathway of these receptors were recently made. The data are intensively discussed elsewhere in this book.

Anti-tumor effects of GnRHa in ovarian, breast and endometrial cancer

Direct inhibitory effects of GnRH agonists and antagonists on the *in vitro* proliferation of human breast cancer cell lines were first demonstrated by Blankenstein and co-workers[28], Miller and co-workers[29] and Eidne and co-workers[21]. More recently, respective data were published by Hershkovitz and co-workers[23] and Palyi and co-workers[24] demonstrating anti-proliferative effects of GnRH antagonists in breast cancer cell lines and the inhibition of stimulatory effects of growth factors. Several groups found direct time- and dose-dependent anti-proliferative effects of GnRH agonists and antagonists on human ovarian cancer cell lines. Involvement of annexin V and epidermal growth factor (EGF)-induced mitogen-activated protein (MAP)-kinase activity has been shown [65, 75, 76][1,18,30,31]. In contrast, other groups failed to detect direct anti-tumor effects of GnRHa or observed them only at very high GnRHa concentrations[32,33].

Ho and colleagues[3] published findings of a biphasic effect of the GnRH agonist triptorelin on the human ovarian cancer cell line IGROV-1. After initial growth stimulation during the first 24 h of incubation, proliferation was inhibited by longer treatment with the agonist. In this setting the mitogenic effect was inhibited by neutralization of insulin-like growth factor (IGF)-II using specific antibodies.

Using human ovarian cancer cell line OV-1063 xenografted into nude mice, Yano and associates[31] demonstrated a significant inhibition of tumor growth by chronic treatment with the GnRH antagonist cetrorelix but not with the agonist triptorelin. As both GnRHa induced a comparable suppression of the pituitary–gonadal axis, the authors speculated that the anti-tumor effects of cetrorelix were exerted directly on GnRH receptors in the tumors. This hypothesis is supported by the *in vitro* data reviewed above. Using another ovarian cancer cell line xenograft (HTOA), Yano and colleagues demonstrated anti-proliferative effects of the GnRH antagonist cetrorelix as well as of the agonist buserelin *in vivo* [76].

In contrast, Manetta and co-workers[33] observed no anti-proliferative effects on ovarian cancer cell lines *in vitro*, but a highly significant effect on the tumor growth of one of these cell lines in nude mice. The authors speculated that the anti-tumor effects of cetrorelix resulted from inhibition of the pituitary–gonadal axis and gonadotropin secretion. Maruuchi and associates[34] supported this hypothesis with *in vitro* inhibition of follicle stimulating hormone (FSH)-induced proliferation of primary rat cancer cell lines by the GnRH agonist buserelin and histopathological tumor regression in this rat model *in vivo*.

Comparable data were published about endometrial carcinomas. Antiproliferative effects and inhibition of stimulatory effects of growth factors of GnRH agonists and antagonists have been shown *in vitro* by several groups [75][4,5,19,24,35]. Others failed to detect these effects or could only find them partly[15,36,37]. Gonadotropin dependence is not supposed to be essential in the growth regulation of endometrial carcinoma.

CYTOTOXIC ANALOGUES OF GnRH

In addition to the mechanisms discussed above, GnRH receptors on tumor cells might also be used for targeted chemotherapy. GnRHa linked covalently to cytotoxic radicals could bind specifically to GnRH receptors with their peptide moiety and act as chemotherapeutic agents after internalization of the ligand–receptor complex into cancer cells or by membrane action. In this fashion, these conjugates could selectively affect those cells that possess GnRH receptors and thus exert fewer side-effects than unconjugated cytotoxic compounds[38]. A great variety of cytotoxic analogues containing different GnRH agonists and antagonists and different cytotoxic compounds including melphalan, cisplatin, methotrexate and cyclophosphamide derivatives have been synthesized in past years[39–42]. Most of these compounds preserved their GnRHa action and were internalized into cells expressing receptors. Major problems, however, were caused by the instability of these compounds in solution and their lack of preservation of their cytotoxic action[42–46].

Now new cytotoxic analogues derived from GnRH analogues, having a D-Lys moiety in position 6, seem to solve these problems. This amino acid offers an amino side chain for convenient attachment of various cytotoxic compounds. Even bulky molecules have been linked to the ε-amino group of the D-Lys^6 moiety, without significant loss of binding affinity of the peptide portion to the receptors for GnRH[46,47]. Recently, encouraging results have been achieved with the cytotoxic analogues AN-152 ([D-Lys^6]-GnRH linked to doxorubicin) and AN-207 ([D-Lys^6]-GnRH linked to 2-pyrrolinodoxorubicin, a derivative of doxorubicin that is 500–1000 times more potent than its parent compound)[47,48]. In rat pituitary cells, AN-207 selectively and reversibly damages gonadotropes[49]. In nude mice with an ovarian carcinoma xenograft expressing GnRH receptors, treatment with AN-207 significantly inhibited tumor growth while the cytotoxic residue alone (2-pyrrolinodoxorubicin) in equivalent doses was toxic to the animals and had no significant effect on tumor growth. Treatment with AN-207 down-regulated receptors for GnRH and decreased EGF receptor levels as well as expression of their mRNA[50]. AN-152 had similar effects in GnRH receptor-positive OV-1063 ovarian cancer cell lines xenografted into nude mice, but no effect on tumor volume in GnRH receptor-negative UCI-107 cell lines was observed[51]. Szepeshazi and co-workers[52] investigated the effects of AN-207 and AN-152 and their respective cytotoxic residues on GnRH receptor-positive MXT mouse mammary tumors: both compounds inhibited tumor growth significantly while their cytotoxic residues alone were toxic to the animals without affecting tumor growth. In addition, in these experiments a decrease in the mitotic index and an increase in apoptosis have been shown after treatment with cytotoxic GnRHa.

In endometrial cancer cell lines the cytotoxic effect of AN-152 was blocked by an excess of GnRH antagonists in the fashion of competitive inhibition, indicating that this cytotoxic GnRHa acts through GnRH receptors[53].

Nechushtan and co-workers[54] published promising data about GnRH linked to the chimeric *Pseudomonas* exotoxin PE66. They found selective anti-tumor activity in a variety of gynecological and other adenocarcinomas. These data suggest a selective receptor-mediated action of cytotoxic analogues of GnRH that could lead to target cell-specific cytotoxic chemotherapy with the possibility of dose intensification and reduction of toxicity.

RESULTS OF RECENT CLINICAL RESEARCH

Breast cancer

The suppression of ovarian steroid synthesis is still accepted as the main mechanism of action of GnRHa in advanced estrogen-dependent breast cancer of pre- and perimenopausal women[55–57]. In early and advanced estrogen-dependent breast cancer the endocrine therapy of first choice is still tamoxifen as the classical anti-estrogen. A main disadvantage of tamoxifen is its stimulatory effects on the ovaries in premenopausal women, possibly by actions on the hypothalamic–pituitary axis blocking the negative feedback regulation of estrogens and resulting in supraphysiological levels of estradiol and in ovarian cysts[55,58]. In addition, the partial estrogen agonist action of tamoxifen may lead to development of endometrial cancer and to stimulation of breast cancer cells[59,60].

The treatment of advanced breast cancer in pre- and perimenopausal women with GnRHa is now widely accepted. Response rates between 31% in unselected and 63% in estrogen receptor-positive cancers have been reported[61–63]. These data were recently confirmed by Untch[64], who reported on an open prospective trial on leuporelinacetate in pre- and perimenopausal women with metastatic breast cancer with an overall response rate of 34% (25 of 73 patients). The largest sample published is pooled data about 228 patients; these had an objective response to goserelin in 36% and a median duration of response of 44 weeks[65].

In 1995, Jonat and associates[66] reported the results of a randomized study comparing the effects of the GnRH agonist goserelin alone or in combination with tamoxifen in 318 pre- and perimenopausal women with advanced breast cancer. In the whole group there was no statistically significant difference in response rates and survival but a benefit in favor of combination therapy regarding time to progression. In the subgroup of patients with skeletal metastases only, significant differences in favor of combination therapy were seen in response rate, time to progression and survival.

Further results have now been presented [47]. The EORTC has performed a meta-analysis collecting data from 506 premenopausal patients randomized between GnRHa (goserelin or buserelin) plus tamoxifen vs. GnRHa alone. The results strongly favored the combination therapy with objective response rates of 39% vs. 30% ($p = 0.03$), median progression-free survival of 8.7 months vs. 5.4 months ($p < 0.001$) and median overall survival of 2.9 years vs. 2.5 years ($p = 0.02$). Jonat proposes the combined treatment modality as a new standard regimen in premenopausal women with advanced breast cancer, suitable for hormonal manipulation [47].

These encouraging results and the good tolerability led to the initiation of trials on GnRHa in the adjuvant setting [48]. These protocols compare GnRHa treatment with standard cytotoxic chemotherapies such as cyclophosphamide, methotrexate and 5-fluorouracil (Zoladex Early Breast Cancer Association (ZEBRA), International Breast Cancer Study Group (IBCSG)) or cyclophosphamide, doxorubicin and 5-fluorouracil (Eastern Co-operative Oncology Group (ECOG), South Western Oncology Group (SWOG)) or endocrine treatment with tamoxifen and the combination of GnRHa with tamoxifen (Cancer Research Campaign (CRC)). Preliminary results will soon be available and may lead to the use of GnRHa in the adjuvant treatment of breast cancer [48][56].

Another indication for GnRHa in breast cancer treatment was presented by Cardamakis [61]. As outlined above, tamoxifen may cause ovarian cysts that can lead to discontinuation of treatment. In 11.6% of postmenopausal women treated with tamoxifen for breast cancer, ovarian cysts were detected. Most of these cysts disappeared after GnRHa treatment so that discontinuation of tamoxifen application or surgical investigation could be avoided [61].

Ovarian cancer

Several studies have been published that were performed to investigate potential beneficial effects of suppression of endogenous gonadotropins by GnRHa in addition to standard cytotoxic chemotherapy. Medl and colleagues[67] treated 15 patients with triptorelin during carboplatin-based standard chemotherapy and for a further 6 months. Compared to a control group of patients treated with chemotherapy alone, there was a positive trend but no statistically significant differences in terms of response, survival and time to progression. Similar data were published by Falkson and co-workers[68]. They treated 34 patients randomized to receive cisplatin alone or cisplatin plus triptorelin and could not achieve significant differences but a positive tendency for the combination. Finally, a prospective, randomized, double-blind multicenter trial was performed. Treatment of 135 patients with stage III or IV epithelial ovarian cancer after cytoreductive surgery with standard platinum-based cytotoxic chemotherapies in combination with or without the GnRH agonist triptorelin showed no significant differences regarding time to progression and overall survival, although a reliable suppression of gonadotropins in the triptorelin-treated group was achieved[69]. It was suggested that the suppression of endogenous gonadotropins by conventional doses of a GnRH agonist produced no relevant beneficial effect in patients with advanced ovarian carcinoma who received standard surgical cytoreduction and cytotoxic chemotherapy[69].

Apart from this, there are certain hints of the efficacy of single-agent hormonal treatment with GnRHa in patients with refractory advanced ovarian cancer[70]. Emons and Schulz[71] reviewed several phase-II studies with altogether 171 patients, observing 21 objective remissions (12%) and 32 stable diseases (19%). The duration of response varied between 26 and 98+ weeks. Miller and associates[72] reported on an additional 25 patients with refractory ovarian cancer treated with triptorelin. They observed one partial remission (4%), and 15 patients (60%) experienced stable disease for at least 8 weeks. De Vries and Bonte[73] obtained two partial remissions and three stable diseases in 14 patients treated with goserelin. Carnino and colleagues[74] reported 14 stable diseases in 20 patients treated with triptorelin for advanced ovarian cancer[74]. Van der Vange and co-workers[75] reported their experience from eight patients with advanced ovarian cancer and no reasonable option of successful cytotoxic chemotherapy. One of the eight patients had a complete remission of a pelvic recurrence (> 5 cm) and of elevated CA 125 levels for more than 38 months. In all of these publications the very good tolerability of GnRHa was emphasized, especially compared to cytotoxic chemotherapy, which is often of very limited efficacy in this situation.

Preliminary data about treatment with GnRH antagonists in advanced ovarian cancer were presented. Seventeen women with advanced ovarian cancer who had been pretreated with several salvage chemotherapies were treated subcutaneously with 10 mg/day of cetrorelix. At this high dose not only can gonadotropin suppression be achieved but the resulting cetrorelix plasma levels are equivalent to the concentrations leading to direct anti-proliferative effects *in vitro*. Out of 17 patients evaluable so far, three have had temporary partial remissions, and two have had stable disease with time to progression between 125 and 196 days compared to a median time to progression of 59 days in the whole group [64].

In conclusion, a combination of GnRHa and cytotoxic chemotherapy seems not to be more efficacious than cytotoxic therapy alone. In advanced and intensively pretreated cases of ovarian cancer GnRH agonists and antagonists might be a useful addition to the therapeutic armamentarium, especially in view of the very good tolerability.

Endometrial cancer

Several years ago, the first papers on the effects of GnRH agonists on endometrial cancer were published. However, to date only small numbers of patients have been treated and no clear judgement on the efficacy of this approach is possible.

In 1991, Gallagher and colleagues[76] reported on 17 patients with advanced endometrial cancer, refractory to surgery, progestins and radiotherapy, who were treated with GnRH agonists (leuprorelin or goserelin). An objective response was achieved in six of 17 patients (35%; one complete remission, five partial remissions). Continuing this trial, Jeyarajah and co-workers[77] treated another 15 patients and reported three additional cases of objective response. In the whole series this produced nine objective responses in 32 patients (28%; two complete remissions, seven partial remissions). Analyzing their data, the authors observed better responses in recurrences that had been irradiated previously. No correlation with previous progestogen exposure was found. De Vries and Bonte[73] treated seven patients, with two responders (28%; no complete remissions, two partial remissions). Covens and associates[78] treated 25 patients with no objective response. Markmann and co-workers[79] treated nine patients and observed no objective response either.

In addition, one case of down-sizing of a low-grade endometrial stromal sarcoma by the combination of megestrol acetate and the GnRH agonist leuprorelin has been reported[80]. The treatment of simple and complex endometrial hyperplasias with GnRH agonists has been shown to be effective[81].

Considering the limited efficacy and severe side-effects of cytotoxic chemotherapy and the high doses of progestogens used in advanced or recurrent endometrial cancer, the use of GnRH agonists deserves further evaluation.

Prevention of ovarian damage by chemotherapy

Blumenfeld reported data suggesting that the application of a GnRHa prevents premature ovarian failure in young women receiving cytotoxic chemotherapies [66]. A total of 43 cycling women receiving cytotoxic chemotherapy for lymphoma, leukemia or non-malignant autoimmune disease were treated in a prospective trial with the GnRH agonist triptorelin and compared to another 40 women treated with chemotherapy for lymphoma. Inhibin A was measured to reflect the ovarian granulosa cell compartment. Whereas all but one of the surviving patients in the GnRHa/chemotherapy co-treatment group resumed spontaneous ovulation and menses within 6 months, only half of the patients in the control group (chemotherapy alone) resumed ovarian function and regular menstrual cycles ($p < 0.05$). Inhibin A may serve as a prognostic factor, as the concentrations decreased during co-treatment and increased to normal levels in the patients who resumed regular ovarian cyclicity.

The authors propose to consider GnRHa co-treatment in every woman of reproductive age receiving cytotoxic chemotherapy, especially because alternative methods such as assisted reproduction and investigational attempts at ovarian cryopreservation for future *in vitro* maturation can hardly be performed as a routine at the moment [66][82–85].

SUMMARY AND FUTURE PERSPECTIVES

GnRH, GnRH receptors and anti-proliferative effects of GnRHa are present in human ovarian, breast and endometrial cancers. It is likely that a GnRH-based autocrine system is present in these malignant tumors. This system is supposed to be responsible for negative autocrine regulation of cancer cell proliferation, interfering with growth factors, growth factor receptors and related oncogene products. Knowledge of the mechanisms of these actions is rapidly growing.

In addition to these direct actions based on physiological receptor signalling mechanisms, GnRH receptors on tumor cells might be used for targeted chemotherapy with GnRHa linked covalently to cytotoxic radicals. Preclinical data available to date suggest a selective receptor-mediated action of new cytotoxic GnRHa that could lead to specific cytotoxic chemotherapy with dose intensification and reduction of general toxicity.

The clinical value of GnRHa in advanced estrogen-dependent premenopausal breast cancer has been proved for some years. The combined treatment modality of a GnRHa plus tamoxifen has been shown to be even more efficacious. This is proposed as a new standard regimen in premenopausal women with advanced breast cancer suitable for hormonal treatment.

These encouraging data and the good tolerability have led to the initiation of a series of trials on GnRHa in the adjuvant setting. The first results are expected soon.

In contrast to the established situation in breast cancer, GnRHa treatment of ovarian and endometrial cancer is still experimental and should be performed only in clinical trials or in cases where no other reasonable therapeutic option is available.

In ovarian cancer, the combination of GnRHa and cytotoxic chemotherapy seems to be no more efficacious than cytotoxic therapy alone. Only in advanced and intensively pretreated cases of ovarian cancer might single-agent GnRH agonist or antagonist treatment be a useful tool, regarding the very good tolerability of GnRHa and the extremely limited efficacy of cytotoxic chemotherapy in this situation. The use of high doses of GnRH antagonists might provide further advantages. In advanced endometrial cancer there are clear hints of the efficacy of GnRHa treatment. Considering the limited efficacy and severe side-effects of cytotoxic chemotherapy or of high doses of progestogens, the use of GnRH agonists certainly deserves further evaluation. Phase-II data suggest a value of GnRHa in preservation of ovarian function in young women receiving cytotoxic chemotherapy for other malignancies. It is hoped that these data will be confirmed by controlled trials.

REFERENCES

1. Emons G, Ortmann O, Schulz K-D. GnRH analogues in ovarian, breast and endometrial cancers. In Lunenfeld B, Insler V, eds. *GnRH Analogues: The State of the Art 1996*. Carnforth, UK: Parthenon Publishing, 1996:95–120
2. Emons G, Ortmann O, Schulz K-D, *et al*. Growth-inhibitory actions of analogues of luteinizing hormone-releasing hormone on tumor cells. *Trends Endocrinol Metab* 1997;8: 355–62
3. Ho MN, Delgado CH, Owens GA, *et al*. Insulin like growth factor-II participates in the biphasic effect of a gonadotropin-releasing hormone agonist on ovarian cancer cell growth. *Fertil Steril* 1997;67:870–6

4. Emons G, Müller V, Ortmann O, et al. Effects of LHRH-analogues on mitogenic signal transduction in cancer cells. *J Steroid Biochem Mol Biol* 1998;65:199–206
5. Imai A, Takagi A, Horibe S, et al. Evidence for tight coupling of gonadotropin-releasing hormone receptor to stimulated Fas ligand expression in reproductive tract tumors: possible mechanism for hormonal control of apoptotic cell death. *J Clin Endocrinol Metab* 1998;83:427–31
6. Imai A, Takagi A, Horibe S, et al. Fas and Fas ligand system may mediate antiproliferative activity of gonadotropin-releasing hormone receptor in endometrial cancer cells. *Int J Oncol* 1998;13:97–100
7. Yin H, Cheng KW, Hwa HL, et al. Expression of the messenger RNA for GnRH and its receptor in human cancer cell lines. *Life Sci* 1998;62:2015–23
8. Seppälä M, Wahlström T. Identification of luteinizing hormone-releasing factor and alpha subunit of glycoprotein hormones in ductal carcinoma of the mammary gland. *Int J Cancer* 1980;26:231–3
9. Bützow R, Huhtaniemi I, Clayton R, et al. Cultured mammary carcinoma cells contain gonadotropin-releasing hormone-like immunoreactivity, GnRH binding sites and chorionic gonadotropin. *Int J Cancer* 1987;39:498–501
10. Harris N, Dutlow C, Eidne K, et al. Gonadotropin-releasing-hormone gene expression in MDA-MB-231 and ZR-75-1 breast carcinoma cell lines. *Cancer Res* 1991;51:2577–81
11. Ohno T, Imai A, Furui T, et al. Presence of gonadotropin-releasing hormone and its messenger ribonucleic acid in human ovarian epithelial carcinoma. *Am J Obstet Gynecol* 1993;169:605–10
12. Irmer G, Bürger C, Müller R, et al. Expression of the messenger RNAs for luteinizing hormone-releasing hormone (LHRH) and its receptor in human ovarian epithelial carcinoma. *Cancer Res* 1995;55:817–22
13. Imai A, Ohno T, Iida K, et al. Presence of gonadotropin-releasing hormone receptor and its messenger ribonucleic acid in endometrial carcinoma and endometrium. *Gynecol Oncol* 1994;55:144–48
14. Irmer G, Bürger C, Ortmann O, et al. Expression of luteinizing hormone-releasing hormone and its mRNA in human endometrial cancer cell lines. *J Clin Endocrinol Metab* 1994;79:916–19
15. Chatzaki E, Bax CM, Eidne KA, et al. The expression of gonadotropin-releasing hormone and its receptor in endometrial cancer, and its relevance as an autocrine growth factor. *Cancer Res* 1996;56:2059–65
16. Eidne KA, Flanagan CA, Harris NS, et al. Gonadotropin-releasing hormone binding sites in human breast carcinoma. *Science* 1985;229:989–91
17. Fekete M, Wittliff JL, Schally AV. Characteristics and distribution of receptors for [D-Trp^6]-luteinizing hormone-releasing hormone, somatostatin, epidermal growth factor and sex steroids in 500 biopsy samples of human breast cancer. *J Clin Lab Anal* 1989;3:137–47
18. Emons G, Ortmann O, Becker M, et al. High affinity binding and direct antiproliferative effects of LHRH analogues in human ovarian cancer cell lines. *Cancer Res* 1993;54:5439–46
19. Emons G, Schröder B, Ortmann O, et al. High affinity binding and direct antiproliferative effects of luteinizing hormone-releasing hormone in human endometrial cancer cell lines. *J Clin Endocrinol Metab* 1993;77:1458–64

20. Paradiso A, Pezzetta A, Cellamare G, et al. GnRH receptors in human breast cancer and its contiguous not-involved breast tissue. *J Endocrinol Invest* 1999;in press
21. Eidne KA, Flanagan CA, Harris NS, et al. Gonadotropin-releasing hormone (GnRH)-binding sites in human breast cancer cell lines and inhibitory effects of GnRH antagonists. *J Clin Endocrinol Metab* 1997;64:425–32
22. Kakar SS, Musgrove LC, Devor DC, et al. Cloning, sequencing, and expression of human gonadotropin-releasing hormone (GnRH) receptor. *Biochem Biophys Res Commun* 1992; 189:289–95
23. Hershkovitz E, Marbach M, Bosin E, et al. Luteinizing hormone-releasing hormone antagonists interfere with autocrine and paracrine growth stimulation of MCF-7 mammary cancer cells by insulin like growth factors. *J Clin Endocrinol Metab* 1993;77:963–8
24. Palyi I, Vincze B, Kalnay A. Effect of gonadotropin releasing hormone analogues and their conjugates on gonadotropin-releasing hormone receptor-positive human cancer cell lines. *Cancer Detect Prev* 1996;20:146–52
25. Pahwa GS, Kullander S, Vollmer G, et al. Specific low affinity binding sites for gonadotropin-releasing hormone in human endometrial carcinomata. *Eur J Obstet Gynecol* 1991; 41:135–42
26. Srkalovic G, Wittliff JL, Schally AV. Detection and partial characterisation of receptors for [D-Trp^6]-luteinizing hormone-releasing hormone and epidermal growth factor in human endometrial carcinoma. *Cancer Res* 1990;50:1841–6
27. Srkalovic G, Schally AV, Wittliff JL, et al. Presence and characteristics of receptors for [D-Trp^6]-luteinizing hormone-releasing hormone and epidermal growth factor in human ovarian cancer. *Int J Oncol* 1998;12:489–98
28. Blankenstein MA, Henkelmann MS, Klijin JMG. Direct inhibitory effect of a luteinizing hormone-releasing hormone agonist on MCF-7 human breast cancer cells. *Eur J Cancer Clin Oncol* 1985;21:1493–9
29. Miller WR, Scott WN, Morris R, et al. Growth of human breast cancer cells inhibited by a luteinizing hormone-releasing hormone agonist. *Nature (London)* 1985;313:231–3
30. Shibata S, Sato H, Karube A, et al. Involvement of annexin V in antiproliferative effects of gonadotropin-releasing hormone agonists on human endometrial cancer cell line. *Gynecol Oncol* 1997;66:217–21
31. Yano T, Pinski J, Radulovic S, et al. Inhibition of human epithelial ovarian cancer cell growth *in vitro* by agonistic and antagonistic analogues of luteinizing hormone-releasing hormone. *Proc Natl Acad Sci USA* 1994;91:1701–5
32. Connor JP, Buller RE, Conn PM. Effects of GnRH analogues on six ovarian cancer cell lines in culture. *Gynecol Oncol* 1994;54:80–4
33. Manetta A, Gamboa-Vujicic G, Paredes P, et al. Inhibition of growth of human ovarian cancer in nude mice by luteinizing hormone-releasing hormone antagonist cetrorelix. *Fertil Steril* 1995;63:282–7
34. Maruuchi T, Sugiyama T, Kataoka A, et al. Effects of a gonadotropin-releasing hormone agonist on rat ovarian adenocarcinoma cell lines *in vitro* and *in vivo*. *Jpn J Cancer Res* 1998;89:977–83
35. Kleinmann D, Roberts CT, LeRoith D, et al. Regulation of endometrial cancer cell growth by insulin-like growth factors and the luteinizing hormone-releasing hormone antagonist SB-75. *Regul Peptides* 1993;48:91–8

36. Kleinmann D, Douvdevani A, Schally AV, et al. Direct growth inhibition of human endometrial cancer cells by the gonadotropin-releasing hormone antagonist SB-75: role of apoptosis. Am J Obstet Gynecol 1994;170:96–102
37. Borri P, Coronello M, Pesciullesi A, et al. Differential inhibitory effects on human endometrial carcinoma cell growth of luteinizing hormone-releasing hormone analogues. Gynecol Oncol 1998;71:396–403
38. Schally AV, Nagy A, Szepeshazi K, et al. LH-RH analogues with cytotoxic radicals. In Filicori M, Flamigni C, eds. Treatment with GnRH Analogs: Controversies and Perspectives. Carnforth, UK: Parthenon Publishing, 1996:33–44
39. Bajusz S, Janaky T, Csernus VJ, et al. Highly potent analogues of luteinizing hormone-releasing hormone containing D-phenylalanine nitrogen mustard in position 6. Proc Natl Acad Sci USA 1989;86:6318–22
40. Janaky T, Juhasz A, Bajusz S, et al. Analogues of luteinizing hormone-releasing hormone containing cytotoxic groups. Proc Natl Acad Sci USA 1992;89:972–6
41. Milovanovic SR, Radulovic S, Schally AV. Evaluation of binding of cytotoxic analogues of luteinizing hormone-releasing hormone to human breast cancer and mouse MXT mammary tumors. Breast Cancer Res Treat 1992;24:147–58
42. Milovanovic SR, Monje E, Szepeshazi K, et al. Effect of treatment with LHRH analogues containing cytotoxic radicals for luteinizing hormone-releasing hormone in MTX mouse mammary carcinoma. J Cancer Res Clin Oncol 1993;119:273–8
43. Pinski J, Yano T, Janaky T, et al. Evaluation of biological activities of new LH-RH antagonists (T-series) in male and female rats. Int J Peptide Protein Res 1993;41:66–73
44. Rekasi S, Szöke B, Nagy A, et al. Effect of luteinizing hormone-releasing hormone analogs containing cytotoxic radicals on the function of rat pituitary cells: tests in a long term superfusion system. Endocrinology 1993;132:1991–2000
45. Szöke B, Horvath J, Halmos G, et al. LH-RH analogue carrying a cytotoxic radical is internalised by rat pituitary cells in vitro. Peptides 1994;15:359–66
46. Schally AV, Nagy A. Chemotherapy targeted to hormone receptors on tumors. Eur J Endocrinol 1999;in press
47. Nagy A, Schally AV, Armatis P, et al. Cytotoxic analogues of luteinizing hormone-releasing hormone containing doxorubicin or 2-pyrrolinodoxorubicin, an analogue 500–1000 times more potent: structure–activity relationship of daunosamine-modified derivates of doxorubicin. Proc Natl Acad Sci USA 1996;93:7269–73
48. Nagy A, Armatis P, Schally AV. High yield conversion of doxorubicin to 2-pyrrolinodoxorubicin, an analogue 500–1000 times more potent: structure–activity relationship of daunosamine-modified derivation of doxorubicin. Proc Natl Acad Sci USA 1996;93:2464–9
49. Kovacs M, Schally AV, Nagy A, et al. Recovery of pituitary function after treatment with a targeted cytotoxic analog of luteinizing hormone-releasing hormone. Proc Natl Acad Sci USA 1997;94:1420–525
50. Miyazaki M, Schally AV, Nagy A, et al. Targeted cytotoxic analogue of luteinizing hormone-releasing hormone AN-207 inhibits growth of OV-1036 human epithelial ovarian cancers in nude mice. Am J Obstet Gynecol 1999;180:in press
51. Miyazaki M, Nagy A, Schally AV, et al. Growth inhibition of ovarian cancers by cytotoxic analogues of luteinizing hormone-releasing hormone. J Natl Cancer Inst 1997;89:1803–9

52. Szepeshazi K, Schally AV, Nagy A, et al. Targeted cytotoxic luteinizing hormone-releasing hormone analogue inhibits growth of estrogen independent MXT mouse mammary cancers *in vivo* by decreasing cell proliferation and inducing apoptosis. *Anticancer Drugs* 1997;8:974–87
53. Westphalen S, Höppker M, Kotulla G, et al. Receptor mediated endocytosis of cytotoxic LH-RH analogue AN-152 in human endometrial cancer cell lines. *Exp Clin Endocrinol Diabetes* 1998;106(Suppl 1):26
54. Nechushtan A, Yarkoni S, Marianovsky I, et al. Adenocarcinoma cells are targeted by the new GnRH-PE66 chimeric toxin through specific gonadotropin-releasing hormone binding sites. *J Biol Chem* 1997;272:11597–603
55. Jonat W. Luteinizing hormone-releasing hormone analogues – the rationale for adjuvant use in premenopausal women with early breast cancer. *Br J Cancer* 1998;78(Suppl 4):5–8
56. Kaufmann M. Luteinizing hormone releasing hormone analogues in early breast cancer: updated status of ongoing clinical trials. *Br J Cancer* 1998;78(Suppl 4):9–11
57. Minckwitz GV, Kaufmann M. New endocrine approaches in the treatment of breast cancer. *Biomed Pharmacother* 1998;52:122–32
58. Baum M. Tamoxifen – the treatment of choice. Why look for alternatives? *Br J Cancer* 1998;78(Suppl 4):1–5
59. Assikis VJ, Neven P, Jordan VC, et al. A realistic clinical perspective of tamoxifen and endometrial carcinogenesis. *Eur J Cancer* 1996;32A:1464–76
60. Katzenellenbogen BS, Montano MM, Ekena K, et al. Antiestrogens: mechanisms of action and resistance in breast cancer. *Breast Cancer Res Treat* 1997;44:23–38
61. Burger CW, Prinssen HM, Kenemanns P. LHRH agonist treatment of breast cancer and gynecological malignancies: a review. *Eur J Obstet Gynecol Reprod Biol* 1996;67:27–33
62. Buzdar AU, Hortobagy G. Update on endocrine therapy for breast cancer. *Clin Cancer Res* 1998;4:527–34
63. Kimmick GG, Muss HB. Endocrine therapy in metastatic breast cancer. *Cancer Treat Res* 1998;94:231–54
64. Untch M. Endokrine Primärtherapie des prä- bzw. perimenopausalen metastasierten Mammakarzinoms mit Leuporelinacetat-Depot. *Zentralbl Gynäkol* 1998;120:284–92
65. Blamey RW, Jonat W, Kaufmann M, et al. Goserelin depot in the treatment of premenopausal advanced breast cancer. *Eur J Cancer* 1992;28A:810–14
66. Jonat W, Kaufmann M, Blamey RW, et al. A randomised study to compare the effect of luteinizing hormone-releasing hormone (LH-RH) analogue goserelin with or without tamoxifen in pre- and perimenopausal patients with advanced breast cancer. *Eur J Cancer* 1995;31A:137–42
67. Medl M, Peters-Engel C, Fuchs G, et al. Triptorelin in combination with carboplatin-containing polychemotherapy for advanced ovarian cancer: a pilot study. *Anticancer Res* 1993;13:2373–6
68. Falkson CI, Falkson HC, Falkson G. Cisplatin versus cisplatin plus [D-Trp^6]- LHRH in the treatment of ovarian cancer: a pilot trial to investigate the effect of the addition of a GnRH analogue to cisplatin. *Oncology* 1996;53:313–17
69. Emons G, Ortmann O, Teichert H-M, et al. Luteinizing hormone-releasing hormone agonist triptorelin in combination with cytotoxic chemotherapy in patients with advanced ovarian carcinoma. *Cancer* 1996;78:1452–60

70. Emons G, Kavanagh JJ. Hormonal interactions in ovarian cancer. *Hematol Oncol Clin North Am* 1999;13:145–61
71. Emons G, Schulz K-D. Growth regulation of epithelial ovarian cancer by hormones, peptide growth factors, and cytokines. In Pasqualini JR, Katzenellenbogen BS, eds. *Hormone Dependent Cancer*. New York: Dekker, 1996:509–39
72. Miller DC, Brady MF, Barrett RJ. A phase II trial of leuprolide acetate in patients with advanced epithelial ovarian carcinoma. *Am J Clin Oncol* 1992;15:125–8
73. De Vries G, Bonte J. Possible role of goserelin, an LH-RH agonist in the treatment of gynaecological cancers. *Eur J Gynaecol Oncol* 1993;14:187–91
74. Carnino F, Iskra L, Fuda G, et al. The treatment of progressive ovarian carcinoma with [D-Trp^6]-LHRH. *Eur J Cancer* 1994;30A:1903–4
75. van der Vange N, Greggi S, Burger CW, et al. Experience with hormonal therapy in advanced epithelial ovarian cancer. *Acta Oncol* 1995;34:813–20
76. Gallagher CJ, Oliver RTD, Oram DH, et al. A new treatment for endometrial cancer with gonadotropin releasing-hormone analogue. *Br J Obstet Gynaecol* 1991;98:1037–1041
77. Jeyarajah AR, Gallagher CD, Blake PR, et al. Long-term follow-up of gonadotropin-releasing hormone analog treatment for recurrent endometrial cancer. *Gynecol Oncol* 1996;63:47–52
78. Covens A, Thomas G, Shaw P, et al. A phase II study of leuprolide in advanced/recurrent endometrial cancer. *Gynecol Oncol* 1997;64:126–9
79. Markman M, Kennedy A, Webster K, et al. Leuprolide in the treatment of endometrial cancer. *Gynecol Oncol* 1997;66:542
80. Scribner DR Jr, Walker JL. Low-grade endometrial stromal sarcoma preoperative treatment with Depo-Lupron and Megace. *Gynecol Oncol* 1998;71:458–60
81. Agorastos T, Bontis J, Vakiani A, et al. Treatment of endometrial hyperplasias with gonadotropin-releasing hormone agonist: pathological, clinical, morphometric, and DNA-cytometric data. *Gynecol Oncol* 1997;65:102–14
82. Blumenfeld Z. Prevention of irreversible chemotherapy induced ovarian damage in young women with lymphoma. *Hum Reprod* 1996;11:1620–6
83. Blumenfeld Z. Prevention of gonadal damage during cytotoxic therapy. *Ann Med* 1997;29:199–206
84. Blumenfeld Z. Inhibin A concentrations in the sera of young women during and after chemotherapy for lymphoma: correlation with ovarian toxicity. *Am J Reprod Immunol* 1998;39:33–40
85. Blumenfeld Z, Avivi I. Trying to preserve ovarian function in the face of chemotherapy. *Fertil Steril* 1999;71:773–5

BIBLIOGRAPHY

Abstracts of relevant papers presented at the 5th International Symposium on GnRH Analogues in Cancer and Human Reproduction

23. GnRH-signal transduction in breast, ovarian and endometrial cancers. G. Emons, C. Gründker, P. Völker, Germany
47. LHRHa+ tamoxifen vs. LHRHa alone – results of an EORTC meta-analysis of studies in premenopausal women with advanced breast cancer. W. Jonat, Germany

48. A review of 'Zoladex' in the treatment of breast cancer. M. Kaufmann, Germany
61. Therapeutic aproach to ovarian cysts with GnRH analogues (goserelin) in tamoxifen-treated postmenopausal patients with breast cancer. E. Cardamakis, G. Argiropoulos, A. Korantzis, *et al.*, Greece
62. GnRH receptors (GnRH-R) in human breast tumor (T) and contiguous 'not involved' breast tissue (NT). A. Paradiso, A. Pezzetta, B. Pelagio, *et al.*, Italy
64. First results of the GnRH-antagonist cetrorelix in patients with ovarian cancer. G. Emons, S. Westphalen, K.-D. Schulz, *et al.*, Germany, USA
65. GnRH reduces endometrial, ovarian and breast cancer cell proliferation via inhibition of growth factor-induced mitogenic signal transduction. C. Gründker, P. Völker, K.-D. Schulz, G. Emons, Germany
66. Preservation of ovarian function in young women undergoing chemotherapy. Z. Blumenfeld, Israel
75. Effects of GnRH agonists on the cell growth of ovarian and endometrial carcinoma cell lines. N. Ohyama, J.X. Qiang, S. Shibata, *et al.*, Japan
76. Inhibition of human epithelial ovarian cancer cell growth *in vivo* and *in vitro* by GnRH analogues. T. Yano, N. Yano, H. Matsumi, H. Jimbo, Y. Taketani, Japan

10
GnRH analogues in the management of prostate cancer and benign prostatic hyperplasia

J. E. Altwein

INTRODUCTION

Androgen deprivation is the mainstay of therapeutic options practiced in prostate cancer. Gonadotropin releasing hormone (GnRH) agonists are an essential part of this form of treatment and may be employed as the only endocrine manipulation or in combination with antiandrogens (in other words, maximal androgen blockade). An extensive review of GnRH agonists in prostate cancer has been published by Labrie[1]. In patients with bone metastases, maximal androgen blockade prolongs life by between 3 and 6 months. The patient with minimal metastatic spread, however, may benefit from this combination for much longer. Apart from being used continuously, maximal androgen blockade may be given intermittently. In locally advanced prostate cancer, GnRH agonists alone or together with antiandrogens are at present being studied in conjunction with radical surgery or definitive irradiation. Whether such a neoadjuvant or adjuvant use postpones the time to progression has not yet been decided. The patient with lymph node metastases seems to benefit from early androgen deprivation in conjunction with radical prostatectomy. The randomized Phase-III Eastern Cooperative Oncology Group Trial has demonstrated the efficacy of immediate androgen deprivation; at a follow-up of 6.8 years, 85% of patients with histologically proven lymph node metastases remained prostatic specific antigen (PSA)-negative versus only 37% of men with delayed onset of androgen deprivation[2].

The GnRH agonists seem to exert their anti-tumor activity not only through chemical castration, but also by acting directly on tumor cells by blocking their GnRH receptors[3,4]. GnRH agonists exert a significant and dose-dependent antiproliferative action on LNCaP and DU-145 cells, and it has been confirmed that these cell lines have GnRH receptors on their cell membranes. Recently, Lamhaszi and colleagues have compared the effect of a GnRH agonist (D-Trp[6]-LH-RH) and the antagonist cetrorelix upon the levels of receptors for GnRH and epidermal growth factor (EGF) and expression of mRNA for these receptors in DU-145 human androgen-independent prostate cancers xenografted into nude mice. Tumor growth was only significantly inhibited by cetrorelix but not by the agonist. The concentration of GnRH receptors was reduced by 22% and 67% after 4 weeks of treatment with the agonist and antagonist, respectively. The concentration of EGF receptors fell by 48% with the agonist; however, with cetrorelix the EGF receptor level dropped by 66%[5].

If these *in vitro* data are studied *in vivo*, two extensive phase-III trials deserve to receive great interest. In the Intergroup Study 0036, leuprolide was tested with and without flutamide in metastatic prostate cancer[6]. In this trial, a survival benefit was demonstrated when the maximal androgen blockade was used, i.e. leuprolide plus flutamide. However, in the Intergroup Trial 0105, the GnRH agonist was replaced by bilateral orchiectomy in patients with metastatic carcinoma of the prostate[7]. In this trial, a survival benefit of the combination of surgical castration with flutamide was not found. One is tempted to speculate that the difference could be related to a different mode of action of surgical castration versus medical castration, i.e. administration of GnRH agonists.

To report on papers presented at the 5th International Symposium on GnRH Analogues in Cancer and Human Reproduction, I have made a subjective selection from the presentations. At the present time, at least 14 preparations of potent GnRH antagonists are under development as well as long-acting GnRH agonists. These will lead to better patient acceptance and an enhanced quality of life; however, one cannot anticipate a new mode of androgen deprivation unless it can be shown that direct action on the tumor cell is dominant.

Benign prostatic hyperplasia is at present infrequently treated by endocrine manipulation. An exception may be the 5α-reductase inhibitor finasteride. Therefore, it was of interest to witness the action of a new GnRH antagonist on benign prostatic obstruction.

GnRH ANALOGUES IN MALE INDICATIONS

GnRH antagonists, which are injected intramuscularly or subcutaneously every 4 weeks, avoid the flare phenomenon of the GnRH agonists. Teverelix is injected subcutaneously as a soluble acetate salt. It was tested in male beagle dogs in a dose of 20 mg. Testosterone suppression to less than 50 ng/dl (in other words, castration level) lasted over 60 days. After an initial burst, there is a constant release of teverelix over 45 days which can be measured in plasma for more than 50 days [78]. In another study, the GnRH antagonist abarelix was studied in a prospective, non-randomized trial in 209 patients with prostatic carcinoma [80]. The indication was not given. A small control group of 33 patients received either the GnRH agonist leuprolide or the GnRH agonist goserelin. Abarelix was injected in a dosage of 100 mg on days 1 and 15 and then every 4 weeks. After 1 week, 76% of the patients had a testosterone level of less than 50 ng/dl versus 0% of the control group receiving leuprolide or goserelin. None of the abarelix-treated men had a testosterone surge; however, a surge was observed in all men receiving the agonists [80]. In the literature, approximately 16% of men treated with GnRH agonist are reported to suffer adverse events due to the testosterone surge. Furthermore, it was noted that, following the 4-weekly injections of GnRH agonists, there were microsurges of testosterone; an alleged lack of androgen suppression was observed in 4%. Abarelix caused no serious adverse events; the occasional mentioning of back pain was considered to be unrelated. In essence, the main advantage of abarelix is the rapid onset of action and the absence of flares. However, it is not yet established whether this translates into a prolonged period of progression-free survival.

In a second uncontrolled trial (phase II), abarelix was given neoadjuvantly 4–12 weeks before brachytherapy or irradiation to 36 patients with prostate cancer. After 4 weeks, the prostate volume was reduced by 22%, and by 35% at 3 months. In 35 out of 36 patients, testosterone levels dropped to less than 50 ng/dl after 2 weeks. Fourteen out of 30 patients followed for recovery showed an increase in testosterone levels to more than 100 ng/dl, after discontinuation of abarelix. This number rose to 30 patients by 3 months after discontinuation of the antagonist [81].

During the development of the GnRH agonists, long-acting compounds have been produced. One example is histrelin, which is implanted subcutaneously into the inner arm, giving a daily release of 60 mg over a period of 2 years. Fifteen patients with a metastatic carcinoma of the prostate and a mean pretreatment PSA of 23 ng/ml were treated with histrelin [79]. To suppress the initial testosterone surge, cyproterone acetate or flutamide was given for a period of 90 days. In the flutamide-exposed patients, initial rises of luteinizing hormone (LH), follicle stimulating hormone (FSH) and testosterone levels were observed. However, after 20 days, LH and testosterone levels were completely suppressed. Bolus injection of GnRH did not raise the suppressed LH and testosterone levels. The PSA level reached its nadir after 56 days. The testosterone suppression was reversible.

The authors [79] commented that at present Medicare pays US$750 million per annum for GnRH agonists.

Another long-acting GnRH agonist is Duros® leuprolide, which is again implanted into the inner arm [84]. A testosterone surge up to 637 ng/dl (depending on the number of implants) was observed. Testosterone castration levels were reached after 2–4 weeks. In the 51 patients studied so far, no serious adverse events have been observed. There were no microsurges in testosterone levels [84].

If prostate cancer patients are given palliative treatment, health-related quality of life is of key importance. The effect of surgical castration upon quality of life was measured in 430 men with advanced carcinoma of the prostate [82]. A total of 385 men were castrated according to Riba and 45 had a total orchiectomy. The quality-of-life measurement instruments were Giessen's Complaint Sheet, a general questionnaire, and the Psychological Well Being Questionnaire of Gross. No prostate cancer-specific or cancer-specific modules were employed. It was noted that approximately a quarter of the patients had complications due to surgical castration. The authors concluded that men less than 75 years of age favor GnRH agonists but, in men beyond this age, there was no difference. In all men, there was a severe impact on their sex life. In a comment to this study, Fowler mentioned that, using Litwin's questionnaire and the Short Form 15 instruments, quality of life did not differ whether the men had a medical or surgical castration.

SPECIAL PROBLEMS RELATED TO THE MANAGEMENT OF PROSTATE CANCER

Intermittent androgen deprivation is an interesting concept; however, there are still no conclusive results. The idea behind the cessation of treatment is to make the tumor cell pre-apoptotic again. This should postpone hormone resistance, enhance survival and quality of life, and reduce costs. In trial EC 201, leuprolide is injected four-weekly plus 250 mg flutamide per day. Patients with a $T_{1-4} N_x M_{1b,c}$ prostate cancer received this maximal androgen blockade for 6 months. Patients with a PSA less than 4 ng/ml are randomized at this point to receive either a continuous maximal androgen blockade or the intermittent treatment. In the latter modality, patients are off treatment until the PSA rises to more than 10 ng/ml or the onset of progression. Then, the treatment is resumed until the PSA falls again to less than 4 ng/ml when the treatment is stopped again. At the present time, 128 patients have been recruited; 81 patients have received 6 months of treatment. Forty-eight of these have been randomized, whereas 33 men were not eligible since their PSA never fell below 4 ng/ml. Six patients had flutamide-related adverse events, six progressed, and three had a protocol violation [86].

It is important to discuss PSA relapse after radical prostatectomy. Zattoni and colleagues reported on a series of 1623 radical prostatectomies in which 7.9% had a PSA relapse, i.e. PSA > 2 ng/ml [87]. In men with a pT_1 cancer, 36 months elapsed before PSA relapse, 23 months in the presence of positive margins and 9 months in the presence of seminal vesicle invasion. After 2 years, men with a pT_{3a} carcinoma of the prostate had a 34% PSA failure and after 3 years a 41% PSA failure. The authors quote a case report presented at the European Association of Urology meeting in 1998: 3 years after radical prostatectomy, a gradual PSA increase with a slow doubling time was observed. At that meeting, the audience gave the following vote as to how treatment should proceed: watchful waiting 27%, irradiation 25%, prostatectomy 20%, androgen deprivation 17%, and other forms of treatment 11%. Zattoni and colleagues concluded that the remaining cancer cells following extracapsular radical prostatectomy are effectively killed with early androgen deprivation.

For the future, prognostic factors for carcinoma of the prostate will be important. With the advent of reverse transcription-polymerase chain reaction (RT-PCR) for PSA, the term 'molecular prognosis' has been coined. Kurek and colleagues [89] stated that the RT-PCR for PSA is positive in 70.3% in patients with a pT_2 carcinoma of the prostate. Problems arise when different methods and different specificities are used. The following markers should be tested to enhance the prognostic power: insulin-like growth factor 1, bcl 2, bax, KAI 1, PSA, prostate specific membrane antigen and macrophage inhibiting factor. At the present time, a priority ranking among these markers of potential prognostic relevance cannot be given.

NEOADJUVANT HORMONAL THERAPY BEFORE RADICAL PROSTATECTOMY OR IRRADIATION

Neoadjuvant treatment has been tested in seven centers. A review and meta-analysis of these trials has been published by Bonney and colleagues[8]. One can conclude at this time that a neoadjuvant androgen ablation is significantly associated with a low pT-stage and negative surgical margins. Whether this translates into a prolonged progression-free survival remains to be seen. In a French phase-III trial, 175 patients were recruited [88]. Eighty-six patients were treated over 3 months with a maximal androgen blockade, whereas 89 patients received an immediate radical retropubic prostatectomy. The neoadjuvantly treated patients experienced a reduction in prostate size of 35%; T_1 patients had a 37% and T_3 patients a 39% reduction in volume. Surgery after hormonal treatment was not technically different. Blood loss during surgery was not different whether neoadjuvant treatment was used or not. Following presurgical treatment, 40% of the patients had one clinical T-stage lower than before. The Gleason scores were identical; however, patients with a direct radical prostatectomy had a margin-positive rate of 54% versus 31% after hormonal pretreatment. The International Prostate Symptom Score 12 months after radical prostatectomy was identical in either arm, as was the score for potency: 10% in the pretreated and 9% in the patients with immediate surgery. Continence at 12 months following surgery was complete in 64 of the neoadjuvantly treated and in 50% of those given immediate surgery. Incontinence occurred in 10% of the hormonally treated patients and in 20% of the patients with direct surgery. The results of this French phase III trial were compared to the RTOG 86.10 trial where patients were neoadjuvantly treated before irradiation. Clinical stages were T_{2b}–T_4 and 471 patients were recruited. Local control was achieved in 29% of those receiving irradiation only versus 54% in the group receiving neoadjuvant treatment plus irradiation, and disease-free survival was 20% longer after neoadjuvant treatment plus irradiation. The number of positive postirradiation biopsies was 21% in the irradiation-only group versus 37% in the neoadjuvant-treated group. In an ensuing debate, it was pointed out that late results are missing so that no firm conclusion can yet be drawn.

Brachytherapy with transperineally applied permanent seeds competes with radical prostatectomy in their capabilities for cure. Stone and colleague [92] studied palladium-103 seeds. With proper patient selection (Gleason score ≤ 6 and PSA < 10 ng/ml), 91% of patients were free from PSA failure at 5 years. The higher the Gleason score, PSA or clinical stage, the lower the success rate. Thus, there is a need for adjuvant irradiation or hormonal treatment. A randomized, prospective phase-III trial comparing brachytherapy with radical prostatectomy is not available. Surrogate parameters to assist in reaching a conclusion are perioperative costs of brachytherapy and radical prostatectomy. In a US population-based survey, the cost of brachytherapy exceeded by far that of radical prostatectomy[9]. When the quality of life is assessed with patients after either procedure, it is far higher in those receiving radical prostatectomy than in those treated with brachytherapy. In a recent study by Bissonette and colleagues[10], patients who had undergone radical prostatectomy appeared to have a better quality of life compared to those having undergone brachytherapy. When voiding function is taken into account, it has been noted that, after seed implantation, patients have initially more irritative and obstructive voiding symptoms, while urinary incontinence is initially worse after surgery. However, after 6 months, there is no significant difference between voiding problems after either form of treatment[11]. Finally, since it has been found that dose escalation improves PSA-free survival, this led many authors to combine seed implantation with conformal radiotherapy. Though this does not affect the gastrointestinal toxicity (10%) or acute genitourinary toxicity (40%), it demonstrates that the indication for brachytherapy as a single treatment modality requires good patient preselection[12].

Maximal or combined androgen blockade has been debated for 26 years. At present, 30 different trials have been devoted to the comparison of maximal androgen blockade and monotherapy for advanced cancer of the prostate, without arriving at a definitive conclusion. In a newly reported study, 150 patients were randomized to receive either leuprorelin plus flutamide versus leuprorelin plus cyproterone acetate over 3 weeks. In the study endpoints of time to progression and survival, no differences were observed. Because of this, it was interesting to find out whether a well-tolerated form of monotherapy would be as effective. In a comparison of 150 mg of bicalutamide per day with goserelin or surgical castration plus nilutamide, it could be demonstrated that the efficacy in both treatment arms was not statistically significant. However, sexual interest was maintained longer in patients treated with bicalutamide [94].

Screening for carcinoma of the prostate is another important issue. Two problems are inherent to the screening controversy: the high prevalence of carcinoma of the prostate in men and the low specifity of PSA. In 1988, the Quebec Prospective Randomized Controlled Trial was initiated[13]. The PSA cut-off used was 3 ng/ml. In the unscreened population of 38 056 men, 137 prostate cancer deaths have been observed as opposed to only five deaths in 8137 screened men. Thus the prostate cancer death rates over an 8-year period are in favor of screening with early treatment, with an odds ratio of 3.25 [91]. The practical problems encountered with mass screening were studied in Germany in 11 650 men. Case finding was 20 times higher than in an ongoing, legal program for early detection of prostate cancer in Germany which does not include PSA testing. A total of 262 prostate cancers were found among those screened. The main problem encountered with PSA-based screening was the high false-positive rate when a PSA value of 4 ng/ml is used as a cut-off [90].

In essence, among the medley of topics concerning carcinoma of the prostate, the GnRH antagonists as well as long-acting GnRH agonists are the most important. Although the desired long-term outcome studies are still unavailable, both forms of treatment are equally promising for palliation or adjuvant therapy. Health-related quality of life based on general, cancer-specific and prostate

GnRH ANTAGONISTS IN BENIGN PROSTATIC HYPERPLASIA

Patients with lower urinary tract symptoms due to benign prostatic obstruction are most likely to benefit from shrinkage of the enlarged gland to remove the obstruction to urinary outflow. In a three-arm study, 79 patients were recruited to receive either placebo or low-dose cetrorelix or cetrorelix with an initial loading dose [85]. The treatment lasted 4 weeks. The follow-up time was at least 3 months. Of the patients treated with cetrorelix, 52–54% had a fall in the IPSS score of more than 30% in comparison to only 32% of men treated with placebo. The improvement in Q_{max} was 3 ml/s versus 2 ml/s in the placebo-treated group. The PSA fell significantly only in the group treated with cetrorelix with initial loading. The percentage of patients who were sexually active at day 8 did not differ significantly among the three treatment arms. Testosterone levels returned to baseline at day 64; sexual activity returned to baseline by day 120. Adverse events were hot flushes, impotence and loss of libido in approximately 20% of the men. From a urologist's point of view, the shrinkage of a large prostate, which has led to an impaired outflow, is certainly a point of concern. The reversibility of endocrine changes under cetrorelix is in favor of such a concept.

REFERENCES

1. Labrie F. GnRH agonists in prostate cancer. In Lunenfeld B, Insler V, eds. *GnRH Analogues. The State of the Art 1993*. Carnforth, UK: Parthenon Publishing, 1993:100–21
2. Messing E, Rochester NY, Manola J, et al. Immediate hormonal therapy vs. observation for node positive prostate cancer following radical prostatectomy and pelvic lymphadenectomy: a randomized phase III Eastern Cooperative Oncology Group/Inter Group Trial. *J Urol* 1999;161:673A
3. Dondi D, Limonta P, Moreti RM, et al. Antiproliferative effects of luteinizing hormone-releasing hormone (LHRH) agonists on human androgen-independent prostate cancer cell line DU 145: evidence for an autocrine-inhibitory LHRH loop. *Cancer Res* 1994;54:4091–5
4. Palyi I, Vincze B, Kalnay A, et al. Effect of gonadotropin-releasing hormone analogs and their conjugates on gonadotropin-releasing hormone receptor positive human cancer cell lines. *Cancer Detect Prevent* 1996;20:146–52
5. Lamharzi N, Halmos G, Jungwirth A. Decrease in the level and mRNA expression of LH-RH and EGF receptors after treatment with LH-RH antagonist cetrorelix in DU-145 prostate tumor xenografts in nude mice. *Int J Oncol* 1998;13:429–35
6. Crawford ED, Eisenberger MA, McLeod DG, et al. A controlled trial of leuprolide with and without flutamide in prostatic carcinoma. *N Engl J Med* 1989;321:419–24

7. Eisenberger M, Blumenstein B, Crawford ED, McLeod D, et al. Bilateral orchiectomy with or without flutamide for metastatic prostate cancer. N Engl J Med 1998;339:1036–42
8. Bonney WW, Sched AR, Timberlake DS. Neoadjuvant androgen ablation for localized prostatic cancer: pathology methods, surgical end points and meta-analysis of randomized trials. J Urol 1998;160:1754–60
9. Optenberg S, Thompson I. Comparative analysis of total perioperative charges of radical prostatectomy and brachytherapy. J Urol 1999;161:44A
10. Bissonette E, Lippert MC, Petroni G, et al. Comparison of quality of life in patients treated by either radical prostatectomy of brachytherapy for clinically localized prostate cancer. J Urol 1999;161:131A
11. Petroni G, Fulmer BR, Theodorescu D. Prospective assessment of voiding function after treatment for localized prostate cancer: comparison of interstitial brachytherapy vs. radical prostatectomy. J Urol 1999;161:1310 A
12. Gejerman G, Richter F, Lanteri V, et al. Does the addition of conformal beam radiotherapy to prostate seed implantation cause significant acute toxicity? J Urol 1999;161:1305 A
13. Labrie F, Cusan L, Gomez J-L, et al. Screening und re-screening des Prostatakarzinoms: Die Quebec Studie. In Faul P, Altwein JE, eds. *Screening des Prostatakarzinoms*. Berlin: Springer, 1995:339–52

BIBLIOGRAPHY

Abstracts of relevant papers presented at the 5th International Symposium on GnRH Analogues in Cancer and Human Reproduction

78. Long-lasting suppression of plasma testosterone by Antarelix®-depot: a sustained release preparation of the superantagonist teverelix. F. Boutignon, H. Touchet, F. Moine, D. Mallardé, S. David, R. Deghenghi, France
79. A long acting implant releasing a GnRH agonist suppresses testosterone for over two years in prostate cancer. I.M. Spitz, B. Chertin, T. Lindenberg, R. Catane, N. Algur, A.J. Moo Young, P. Kuzma, A. Farkas, Israel and USA
80. Abarelix-depot (A-D), a potent GnRH pure antagonist in patients (pts) with prostate cancer (PrCA): initial clinical results and endocrine comparison with superagonists Lupron® (L) and Zoladex® (Z). M.B. Garnick, K. Tomera, M. Campion, B. Kuca, M. Gefter, USA
81. Abarelix, a novel and potent GnRH antagonist, induces a rapid and profound prostate gland volume reduction (PGVR) and androgen suppression before brachytherapy (BT) or radiation therapy (XRT). M.B. Garnick, M. Campion, M. Gittelman, B. Kuca, M. Gefter, USA
82. Quality of life under different modalities of androgen-deprivation in advanced prostate cancer. G. Ludwig, W. Ohlig, H.J. Berberich, M. Steiger, Germany
84. Duros™ leuprolide implantable therapeutic system in patients with advanced prostate cancer: one-year results of a phase I/II dose ranging study. J. Fowler, J. Gottesman, The Duros™ Leuprolide Implant Study Group, USA
85. Cetrorelix in the treatment of BPH. Y. Schnaars, H. Riethmüller-Winzen, Germany
86. Intermittent versus continuous hormone deprivation in metastatic prostate cancer: preliminary data of an ongoing European study. N. Mottet, France
87. Immediate or deferred hormone ablation in PSA relapse after radical prostatectomy. F. Zattoni, C. Valotto, S. Bierti, Italy

88. Is there a place for neoadjuvant hormonal therapy before radical prostatectomy or radiation therapy in the management of prostate cancer? P. Teillac, France
89. Will modern molecular methods such as RT-PCR improve the prediction of prognosis in prostate cancer patients? R. Kurek, H. Renneberg, G. Aumüller, U.W. Tunn, Germany
90. Results of a screening program for early detection of early prostate cancer in Germany. J.E. Altwein, Germany
91. Screening decreases prostate cancer death: first analysis of the 1988 Quebec prospective randomized controlled trial. F. Labrie, B. Candas, A. Dupont, L. Cusan, J.-L. Gomez, R.E. Suburu, P. Diamond, J. Levesque, A. Belanger, Canada
92. Prostate brachytherapy: treatment strategies for localized and locally advanced disease. N.N. Stone, R.G. Stock, USA
94. Can combined androgen blockade treatment of metastatic prostate cancer be challenged by monotherapy using bicalutamide 150 mg? R.O. Fourcade, C. Chatelain, D. Haguenauer, France

Index

abarelix,
    depot formulation of, 41
    effect on LH inhibition, 32
    inadvertent administration during pregnancy, 76
    lack of flare-up after, 123
    long-term suppression of testosterone by, 33, 36
    single cf. multiple administrations, 37
    single administration cf. multiple doses, 37
    structure, 32, 35
    sustained-release formulation of, 36
    testosterone suppression by, 123
add-back therapy, 74, 78
    in endometriosis, 100
    use in uterine fibroids, 96
administration,
    development of GnRH agonist protocols, 66–67
    dose-finding studies for controlled ovarian hyperstimulation using cetrorelix and ganirelix, 50
    drug delivery as microgranules, 34
    gel formation, 31, 40
    minimal acceptable delivery profiles, 36
    optimal doses, 38
    orally active antagonist, 41
    sustained-release formulation of abarelix, 36
    technical difficulties with implementation of GnRH antagonists, 31
androgen deprivation as therapy for prostate cancer, 121
antiandrogens, use in sex offenders, 85
antiestrogens, use in uterine fibroids, 97
antiprogestogens, use in uterine fibroids, 97
apoptosis, role of GnRH analogues in, 17
arachidonic acid, role in GnRH action, 10
assisted reproduction,
    GnRH antagonists in, 47–61
    safety of GnRH analogue use in, 77
    use in infertile endometriosis patients, 102, 103

azaline B,
    clinical investigations with, 38–42
    controlled release formulation of, 40
    effect on LH inhibition, 32
    gel formation by, 33, 40
    structure, 32
    suppression of estradiol by, 39
    suppression of testosterone by, 33, 39

Bcl-2 protein, presence in uterine fibroids, 92
benign prostatic hyperplasia, 121–128
bicalutamide, 127
bone mineral density, 74
brachytherapy, 126
brain, GnRH receptors in, 13
breast,
    GnRH function in, 7
    GnRH receptors in, 12
breast cancer, 1
    advanced, 109, 110
    anti-tumor effects of GnRH analogues in, 107
    GnRH analogues,
        for early, 2
        in combination with chemotherapy agents, 110
        use in, 105–114
    GnRH binding sites in, 13
    GnRH receptor expression in, 106
    tamoxifen, 109
buserelin,
    cf. cetrorelix for controlled ovarian hyperstimulation, 55
    cf. cetrorelix in assisted reproduction, 78
    cf. ganirelix for controlled ovarian hyperstimulation, 54
    cf. ganirelix in assisted reproduction, 78
    effect in ovarian cancer, 107
    effect on apoptosis, 18
    first use in IVF, 66
    structure, 66
    use in advanced breast cancer, 110
    use in endometriosis, 101

calcium channels, mobilization of and GnRH
  receptors, 8
cancer,
  anti-proliferative effects of GnRH analogues
    in, 16
  GnRH expression by, 14
  molecular mechanisms mediating anti-tumor
    effects of GnRH, 15
  pituitary cf. peripheral, 17
castration,
  surgical,
    cf. medical, 1
    in sex offenders, 84
    quality of life after, 124
cetrorelix,
  characteristics of, 49
  direct effects of in controlled ovarian
    hyperstimulation, 59
  dose-finding studies for controlled ovarian
    hyperstimulation,
      multiple-dose protocol, 50
      single-dose protocol, 53
  effect in ovarian cancer, 107
  effect of inadvertent administration during
    pregnancy, 76
  effect on apoptosis, 18
  effect on growth factors, 16
  effect on ICSI outcomes and dosage, 52
  effect on IVF cf. ICSI outcomes, 58
  effect on LH inhibition, 32
  effect on ovarian cancer, 14
  epidermal growth factor receptor response
    to, 122
  follicular fluid levels of, 59
  phase III studies of for controlled ovarian
    hyperstimulation, 55, 57
  plasma levels of, 59
  pregnancy rate after use in assisted
    reproduction, 78
  structure, 32
  suppression of LH by, for controlled ovarian
    hyperstimulation, 51
  use in advanced ovarian cancer, 112
  use in assisted reproduction, 47–61
  use in benign prostatic hyperplasia, 128
  use in uterine fibroids, 97
chemotherapy,
  doxorubicin linkage with GnRH analogues
    for, 108
  prevention of ovarian damage by GnRH
    agonists during, 75, 113

side-effects of cytotoxic agents cf. GnRH
  analogues, 113
use of GnRH analogues in combination
  with, 110, 111
contraception (hormonal),
  use in endometriosis, 100
  use in uterine fibroids, 97
  uterine fibroids and, 95
controlled ovarian hyperstimulation,
  future developments in using GnRH antag-
    onists, 61
  GnRH agonists for, 47
  GnRH antagonists for, 49
  short cf. long protocols for, 48
cross-talk between signal cascades, 12
cyproterone acetate, use in sex offenders, 85
cytogenetics of uterine fibroids, 93

danazol, use in endometriosis, 100
doxorubicin, linkage with GnRH analogues for
  chemotherapy, 108

endometrial cancer, 1
  advanced, 112
  GnRH analogue use in, 105–114
  GnRH binding sites in, 13
  GnRH receptor expression in, 106
  use of doxorubicin-linked GnRH analogues
    for, 109
endometriosis, 1, 99–104
  definition and diagnosis of, 99
  estradiol levels for therapy of, 38
  GnRH analogues cf. progestins for, 101
  importance of early diagnosis for treatment
    options, 100
  patient management, 101, 102
    for infertility, 102, 103
  recurrence, 100, 101
  surgery cf. medical therapy, 100
  treatment options, 100
    in infertility, 68
endometrium, GnRH function in, 7
endoscopy, use in endometriosis, 100
epidermal growth factor,
  mitogenic effect of, 15
  response of receptors to cetrorelix, 122
  role in anti-tumor effects, 107
  role in development of uterine fibroids, 92
estradiol,
  decrease in and bone mineral density
    reduction, 74

levels required for therapy of endometriosis and uterine fibroids, 38
suppression of by azaline B, 39

Fas, role in apoptosis, 17
FE200486,
   cf. abarelix, 38
   effect on LH inhibition, 32
   long-term suppression of testosterone by, 33
   structure, 32
flare-up, 66
   GnRH agonist use avoids, 7
   of testosterone levels, 123
   prevention of, 75
   problems of, 75
follicle stimulating hormone (FSH),
   response to GnRH agonists, 66
   response to GnRH antagonists in controlled ovarian hyperstimulation, 49
   role of GnRH in synthesis and release of, 7
   total suppression of, 4

G-protein, 8, 17
ganirelix,
   characteristics of, 49
   depot formulation of, 41
   dose-finding studies for controlled ovarian hyperstimulation, multiple-dose protocol, 53
   effect on LH inhibition, 32
   follicular fluid levels of, 59
   long-term suppression of testosterone by, 33
   phase III studies of for controlled ovarian hyperstimulation, 54
   plasma levels of, 59
   pregnancy rate after use in assisted reproduction, 78
   structure, 32
   use in assisted reproduction, 47–61
GnRH (gonadotropin releasing hormone),
   activity in breast cancer, 106
   activity in endometrial cancer, 106
   activity in ovarian cancer, 106
   autocrine/paracrine role, 7
   binding sites in cancers, 13
   cross-talk between signal cascades induced by, 12
   development of stable analogues for use in ovulation induction, 65
   expression by cancers, 14
   hypophysiotropic actions of, 7
   linked to *Pseudomonas* exotoxin for cytotoxicosis, 109
   mechanism of action, 7–18
   molecular mechanisms mediating anti-tumor effects of, 15
GnRH agonists,
   anti-tumor effects of, 107
      in prostate cancer, 121
   bone mineral density reduction and, 74
   cf. antagonist availability, 3
   cf. antagonists,
      in infertility treatments, 69–71
      in ovarian cancer, 14
      mechanism of action, 48
      structure, 48
   cf. GnRH antagonists, 3
   development of protocols, 66
   effect on myometrial proliferation, 93
   effect on reproductive tissues, 76
   local effects, 1
   long-acting formulations, 123, 124
   positive effects of, 73
   use for controlled ovarian hyperstimulation, 47
GnRH analogues,
   anti-proliferative effects of in cancer, 16
   anti-tumor effects of, 14
   cf. progestins in endometriosis, 101
   cytotoxic variants, 108
   future developments in, 31–44
   future uses in cancer, 113
   long-term treatment of uterine fibroids with, 96
   mechanism of action, 1
   molecular biology, 1
   ovarian cyst therapy during tamoxifen administration, 111
   pharmacological reasons for their use in cancers, 105
   pretreatment of uterine fibroids before surgery, 95
   repeat use in recurrent endometriosis, 101
   role in apoptosis, 17
   role in endometriosis therapy, 99–104
   safety aspects, 73–79
   use in benign prostatic hyperplasia, 121–128
   use in breast cancer, 105–114
   use in combination with chemotherapy agents, 110
   use in combination with tamoxifen, 110
   use in endometrial cancer, 105–114

use in infertile endometriosis patients for
    IVF, 102, 103
use in ovarian cancer, 105–114
use in prostate cancer, 121–128
use in treatment of sex offenders, 83–88
GnRH antagonists,
    action on GnRH receptors, 7
    anti-tumor effects of, 107
    cf. agonists,
        in infertility treatments, 69–71
        in ovarian cancer, 14
        mechanism of action, 48
        structure, 48
    cf. GnRH agonists, 3
    effect on reproductive tissues, 76
    future developments in controlled ovarian
        hyperstimulation using, 61
    history of development, 31
    long-acting formulation of, 38
    pituitary response preservation under treatment with, 60
    technical difficulties with their implementation, 31
    use for controlled ovarian hyperstimulation, 49
    use in advanced ovarian cancer, 112
    use in assisted reproduction, 47–61
    use in benign prostatic hyperplasia, 128
    use in uterine fibroids, 97
GnRH receptors,
    action of GnRH antagonists on, 7
    activation of phospholipase pathway at, 8
    cloning of, 42
    description, 8
    expression in breast cancer, 106
    expression in endometrial cancer, 106
    expression in ovarian cancer, 106
    in extra-pituitary tissues, 12
    molecular mechanisms of signalling, 9
    presence of, 7
    types of, 13
gonadotropin (human menopausal), use in assisted reproduction, 47
goserelin,
    effect on growth factors, 16
    structure, 66
    use in advanced breast cancer, 110
    use in advanced endometrial cancer, 112
    use in advanced ovarian cancer, 111
Gq-proteins, 8
granulosa cells, GnRH function in, 7

granulosa-luteal cells, GnRH receptors in, 12
growth factors, mitogenic effect of, 15

histrelin, 66, 123
hot flushes, 74, 78, 96

incontinence after prostatectomy cf.
    brachytherapy, 126
infertility,
    GnRH agonists for, 2
    GnRH antagonists cf. agonists, 69–71
    patient management in endometriosis, 102, 103
    use of GnRH analogues in, 65–71
inositol phosphate pathway, 8
insulin-like growth factor,
    mitogenic effect of, 15
    role in anti-tumor effects, 107
    role in development of uterine fibroids, 93
intracytoplasmic sperm injection (ICSI),
    outcomes on cetrorelix, 58
    and dose used, 52
intrauterine insemination (IUI), use in infertile
    endometriosis patients, 102
in vitro fertilization (IVF),
    first use of buserelin in, 66
    outcomes on cetrorelix, 58
    use in infertile endometriosis patients, 102

leiomyomatosis peritonealis disseminata, 91
leukemia, GnRH agonists protect ovarian
    function during chemotherapy for, 75
leuprolide,
    effect on reproductive tissues, 76
    structure, 66
    use in prostate cancer, 122
leuprorelin,
    use for maximal androgen blockage, 127
    use in advanced endometrial cancer, 112
    use in endometriosis, 101
    use in sex offenders, 86
luteinizing hormone (LH),
    inhibition by azaline B, 38
    levels in polycystic ovarian syndrome, 68
    prevention of surge by GnRH antagonists
        cf. agonists, 69–70
    response to cetrorelix in controlled ovarian
        hyperstimulation, 51
    response to ganirelix in controlled ovarian
        hyperstimulation, 53
    response to GnRH agonists, 66

role of GnRH in synthesis and release of, 7
suppression by GnRH antagonists, 32
total suppression of, 4
lymphoid cells, GnRH function in, 7
lymphoma, GnRH agonists protect ovarian function during chemotherapy for, 75

medroxyprogesterone acetate,
    use in sex offenders, 86
    uterine fibroids and, 95
microgranules,
    as a drug delivery system, 34
    cumulative release of Antarelix® from, 35
mitogen-activated protein, role in anti-tumor effects, 107
mitogen-activated protein kinase, role in GnRH action, 10
mitogenesis, signal transduction pathway of, 15
myometrium,
    GnRH function in, 7
    proliferation and GnRH agonists, 93
    response to ovarian hormones and development of uterine fibroids, 92

ovarian cancer, 2
    advanced, 111, 112
    buserelin and, 107
    cetrorelix and, 107
    GnRH analogue use in, 105–114
    GnRH binding sites in, 13
    GnRH receptor expression in, 106
    response to GnRH antagonist cf. agonist, 14
    triptorelin and, 107
    triptorelin in combination with chemotherapy agents, 111
    use of doxorubicin-linked GnRH analogues for, 108, 109
ovarian cysts in breast cancer treatment, 110
ovary,
    damage to by chemotherapy, 113
    GnRH function in, 7
    GnRH receptors in, 12, 13
ovulation induction, 1
    development of GnRH agonists protocols for, 67
    development of stable GnRH analogues for use in, 65

pancreatic cancer, GnRH binding sites in, 13
phospholipase C, role in GnRH signal transduction, 15

phospholipase pathway, 8
pituitary, preservation of responses under GnRH antagonist treatment, 60
pituitary cancer, GnRH signal transduction in cf. peripheral cancer, 17
placenta, 7, 12
polycystic ovarian syndrome,
    choice of treatment protocol for in infertility, 68
    in precocious puberty, 75
precocious puberty, 1
    long-term safety of GnRH analogues in, 4
    side-effects of GnRH agonists in, 75
pregnancy,
    GnRH analogue levels and fetal well-being, 4
    inadvertent administration of GnRH agonists during and outcome, 76
    inadvertent administration of GnRH antagonists during and outcome, 76
progestins, use in endometriosis, 100
programmed cell death, see apoptosis
prostate, GnRH function in, 7
prostate cancer, 1
    abarelix in, 123
    androgen deprivation as therapy, 121
    GnRH analogues in, 121–128
    GnRH binding sites in, 13
    histrelin in, 123
    incontinence after prostatectomy cf. brachytherapy, 126
    intermittent androgen deprivation for, 124
    leuprolide in, 122
    management of, 2, 124
    neo-adjuvant hormone therapy prior to prostatectomy, 2
    neoadjuvant hormonal therapy before prostatectomy, 125
    quality of life in, 124
    relapse and prognostic factors, 125
    screening for, 127
    surgical castration cf. GnRH analogues, 2
protein kinase C, 9, 15
Pseudomonas exotoxin, 109
psychotherapy in sex offenders, 84
psychotropic drugs, use in sex offenders, 86

quality of life, 124

RU486, use in uterine fibroids, 97

safety, 41, 73–79
    adverse effects of GnRH analogues on reproductive tissues, 76
    future developments and, 78
    in precocious puberty, 4
    in pregnancy, 4
    inadvertent administration during pregnancy, 76
    of use in assisted reproduction, 77
selective serotonin reuptake inhibitors, use in sex offenders, 85
sex offenders,
    definition of disorders in, 83
    treatment methods for, 83, 84
    treatment of with GnRH analogues, 83–88
side-effects,
    bone mineral density reduction, 74
    in precocious puberty, 75
    of cetrorelix use in uterine fibroids, 97
    of cytotoxic agents cf. GnRH analogues, 113
    of GnRH analogues, 73–79
sleep disturbance, 74, 78
smoking, uterine fibroids and, 95
surgery,
    adjunctive therapy, 2
    castration, quality of life and, 124
    endometriosis, cf. medical therapy, 100
    neoadjuvant hormonal therapy before prostatectomy, 125
    uterine fibroids,
        choices of for, 96
        pretreatment with GnRH analogues before, 95
sweating, 74, 78

T98475, 42, 43
tamoxifen,
    in combination with GnRH analogues, 110
    ovarian cysts and, 110
    use in breast cancer, 109
    use in uterine fibroids, 97
testis,
    GnRH receptors in, 12, 13
testosterone,
    long-term suppression of by abarelix, 33, 36
    long-term suppression of by Antarelix®, 34, 35
    long-term suppression of by azaline B, 33
    long-term suppression of by FE200486, 33
    long-term suppression of by ganirelix, 33
    maximal androgen blockage protocols, 127
    need for suppression of in prostate cancer, 121
    response to GnRH agonists, 66
    suppression by abarelix, 123
    suppression by leuprolide cf. goserelin, 123
    suppression by teverelix, 122
    suppression of by azaline B, 39
teverelix,
    cumulative release *in vitro* from microgranules, 35
    long-term suppression of testosterone by, 34
    structure, 32
    testosterone suppression by, 122
triptorelin,
    cf. cetrorelix in assisted reproduction, 78
    effect in ovarian cancer, 107
    effect on growth factors, 16
    in combination with chemotherapy agents, 111
    in ovarian cancer, 14
    use for ovarian protection during chemotherapy, 113
    use in endometriosis, 101
    use in sex offenders, 86
trophoblast, GnRH receptors in, 13

uterine fibroids, 1, 91–98
    antiestrogens for, 97
    antiprogestogens for, 97
    clinical features of, 94
    cytogenetics of, 93
    estradiol levels for therapy of, 38
    GnRH antagonists for, 97
    growth of, 91
    histogenesis of, 91
    long-term treatment with GnRH analogues, 96
    molecular biology of, 92
    pretreatment with GnRH analogues before surgery, 95